D0974239

Other Harvard Medical School Books published
by Simon & Schuster

Harvard Medical School Family Health Guide
by the Harvard Medical School

Six Steps to Increased Fertility
by Robert L. Barbieri, M.D.; Alice D. Domar, Ph.D.; and
Kevin R. Loughlin, M.D.

The Arthritis Action Program
by Michael E. Weinblatt, M.D.

Healthy Women, Healthy Lives
by Susan E. Hankinson, Sc.D.; Graham A. Colditz, M.D.;
JoAnn E. Manson, M.D., and Frank E. Speizer, M.D.

Eat, Drink, and Be Healthy
by Walter C. Willett, M.D.

The Sensitive Gut
by Harvard Medical School

A Harvard Medical School Book

The Aging Eye

A Fireside Book
Published by Simon & Schuster
New York   London   Toronto   Sydney   Singapore

Rockefeller Center
1230 Avenue of the Americas
New York, NY 10020

For information about special discounts for bulk purchases,
please contact Simon & Schuster Special Sales:
1-800-456-6798 or business@simonandschuster.com

Designed by William Ruoto

Manufactured in the United States of America

10 9 8 7 6 5 4 3 2 1

Library of Congress Cataloging-in-Publication Data

The aging eye : a Harvard Medical School book.
       p.   cm.
Includes bibliographical references.
1. Geriatric opthalmology. 2. Vision disorders in old age. 3. Eye—Aging.
I. Harvard Medical School.
RE48.2.A5 A355 2001
618.97'77—dc21
2001040894
ISBN 0-7432-1503-6

Harvard Medical School gratefully acknowledges Sandra Gordon, the writer of this work; our faculty consultant, B. Thomas Hutchinson, M.D., Associate Clinical Professor of Ophthalmology, Harvard Medical School, Editorial Board, *The Harvard Health Letter;* and Jeffrey S. Heier, M.D. (HMS Appt), Clinical Instructor of Ophthalmology, Harvard Medical School, President, Center for Eye Research and Education, Ophthalmic Consultants of Boston, for his help in reviewing parts of the book.

Contents

Introduction

What's the first thing you do when you sit down to read a magazine or book? If you've reached midlife or beyond, you probably grab your reading glasses. And, if you don't need them yet: get ready. By age sixty-five, you probably will. By then, nearly everyone's eyes feel some effect of aging.

As does the rest of your body, your eyes naturally change throughout your life. But as you get older, the effects become more apparent as the tissues and normal drainage apparatus in your eyes become less efficient. A shift in closeup vision is one of the first problems you're likely to encounter, starting at about age forty. Suddenly, you may notice that you can't see the crossword puzzle as well as you used to, without holding it at arm's length; find it difficult to thread a needle; or, maybe you have trouble focusing in dim light. Although these changes may seem to appear overnight, they actually take years to develop. The good news: These age-related eye problems can be solved with corrective lenses.

However, more serious age-related vision problems may result in vision loss or distortion, which can take on many different forms and may require extensive treatment. Some people see everything in a blur, in double, or through a haze. Others see everything except what's right before them, or they see only what's in front of them, but nothing to either side. Though the symptoms vary in both character and severity, the ultimate consequences are often the same: difficulty performing day-to-day activities, such as reading a newspaper, watching television, doing finances, cooking meals, or crossing the street. Poor vision can dim your quality of life.

One out of every five people is affected by impaired vision by age sixty-five. According to Prevent Blindness America, more than 86 million Americans age forty and above are visually impaired and/or *legally blind*—possessing 20/200 vision or less, with eyeglasses. Each year, an additional 47,000 Americans become totally blind—a tragedy that robs them of joy and independence, and adds to the staggering $4 billion that society spends annually in blindness-related costs. However, you don't have to become a statistic.

EYE OPENER

As the nation's 76 million baby boomers reach older adulthood, it's estimated that twice as many people will be blind by the year 2030 as there are now.

Safeguard Your Sight

There's a lot you can do to protect your vision, now and in the future. It's estimated that at least one-third of the new cases of blindness, for example, could have been averted with preventive care and early diagnosis. Many eye diseases can be reversed or prevented from progressing when they're detected in their early stages.

Unfortunately, many of us aren't as conscientious about caring for our eyes as we are about our other body parts. People tend to take their eyes for granted unless there's a problem, such as blurred vision, redness or pain. However, ask people which of their senses they're most afraid of losing and chances are the majority will say *sight*. Nonetheless, despite reminders to get regular eye exams, we often neglect to visit an ophthalmologist. A regular eye exam is the only way to find an eye disease that has no early signs— by the time symptoms do become obvious, it can be too late for treatment.

What's Included in *The Aging Eye*

To help protect your vision now and in the future, this book discusses three common eye disorders that pose the greatest threat to your vision in the later part of life: cataract, glaucoma, and age-related macular degeneration (AMD). The following pages will help you determine whether you are at risk of developing these disorders, describe their symptoms, and discuss diagnosis and the latest treatments. In addition to these conditions, *The Aging*

Eye also covers conditions common to aging, including presbyopia, dry eye syndrome, floaters and flashes, and retinal detachment. Throughout this book, you'll also gain insight about practical preventive measures that can help you maintain and preserve your vision.

To help you learn how to take the very best care of your eyes as you get older, *The Aging Eye* covers all the bases. Maybe you've never really thought about how your eyes work and the miracle of vision—in chapter 1, you'll take a tour of the eye and get a good idea of how the eye does its job of focusing and converting light into visual images.

Chapter 2 discusses the external and internal changes you can expect to occur through the years. While you can't turn back the clock, you can often compensate for some of the visual decline associated with getting older.

Chapter 3 explains the eye examination in detail. Here, you'll learn what really goes on in a routine eye examination—from testing your vision to inspecting the back of your eye—and why this exam is so important to maintaining your eyesight.

In chapter 4, you'll learn about cataracts—what causes them, what symptoms to watch for, how they're diagnosed and treated, and what to expect after cataract surgery, one of the most common surgeries performed in the United States today.

Chapter 5 covers glaucoma, usually an age-related eye condition, which results from too much fluid pressure inside the eye; in its early stages, it often progresses without symptoms. If left untreated, it can lead to vision loss and blindness.

Age-related macular degeneration is discussed in chapter 6; it's the leading cause of legal blindness among Americans sixty-five and older. Damage caused by the disease can't be reversed, but early detection may help slow its progress. In some cases, it can be treated with laser therapy.

Chapter 7 discusses other common later-life eye disorders, including *presbyopia*—the slow loss of the ability to see close objects or small print, a normal process that happens over a lifetime. Also discussed are eyelid problems, such as *ptosis* (drooping eyelids) and dry eyes, a condition in which tear glands stop either making enough tears, or make tears that are of poor quality. *Floaters* and *flashes*—tiny spots or single flashes of light that appear in your field of vision— are also covered, as is *retinal detachment*, a serious condition in which the inner and outer layers of the *retina*, the thin lining at the back of the eye, separates from its supporting tissue.

There's a lot you can do to prevent or correct eye diseases and conditions. Building on chapters 1 through 7, chapter 8 offers practical suggestions as to what you can do now to preserve your vision, from fine-tuning your diet and stopping smoking, to wearing sunglasses to protecting your eyes from the ravages of diabetes.

Vision naturally changes throughout life, but it's possible to grow older—into your eighties and beyond—with good vision. While older people tend to have more eye problems than do younger people, many eye disorders can be prevented or corrected if you visit your eye doctor.

Don't be blindsided by eye disease. *The Aging Eye* can provide the knowledge you need to safeguard your sight.

In the event of eye disease, it can help you make educated decisions with your ophthalmologist regarding your treatment and care. After all, when it comes to protecting and preserving your vision, especially as you get older, there's no substitute for solid information from a reputable source.

1

How the Eye Works

Without a doubt, sight is a complex and fascinating phenomenon. Almost magically, the eye constantly adjusts the amount of light it lets in, focuses on objects—whether they're at your fingertips or off in the distance—and instantly transmits light to the brain, where it's converted to images. To understand how your eyes and your eyesight change with age, it's helpful to know how your eyes function. Maybe you know a little about the inner workings of the eye because you were diagnosed as nearsighted or farsighted when you were younger. Chances are, however, that unless you've had trouble seeing at some point in your life or had an eye injury, you haven't given your eyes a second thought. To help you better understand your eyes, and how best to maintain and enhance your vision, here's a basic primer on eyesight.

Vision 101

The eye is often compared to an autofocus camera but, in truth, the organ of sight is far more complex and efficient. Not only does the eye focus and snap pictures, it also works continuously with the brain and the nervous system to process everchanging images, and to provide the visual information you need to do everything from hitting a golf ball to preparing your taxes.

Eyeball Engineering: Anatomy and Physiology of the Eye

Despite its reputation as a delicate organ, the eye is remarkably resilient and hardy, engineered by nature to last from infancy through old age. Shaped like a sphere, the eyeball is slightly more than an inch in diameter, with a slight protrusion in front. It sits in a bony, protective socket of the skull, called the *orbit*, and is surrounded by a cushiony layer of fat, fibrous tissue, and muscles.

Eyelids and Eyelashes: The Cleaning Crew

The eyelids and eyelashes have their own unique functions. They act like streetsweepers, keeping a uniform, smooth tear filter on the surface of the eye. The lids constantly brush and blink away dust and other debris that might otherwise blow into the eye. Lining the inner surfaces of the eyelids and the *sclera*, the visible white portion of your eye, is the *conjunctiva*, a thin, colorless membrane that's so sensitive that, when threatened by outside invaders, such as dust or dirt, it automatically triggers a protective reaction—tearing and/or blinking.

Tears course over the surface of the eye and keep it lubricated, well nourished, and clear of foreign matter. They're produced by the *lacrimal* (tear) gland, located behind the upper lid. Tears drain off into the nose through ducts at the innermost corner of the eye. (*See* Figure 1.)

The Extraocular Muscles: Movement Managers

Six muscles, external to the eye but attached to the surface (the *extraocular* muscles), regulate each eye's up-and-down and side-to-side motions. The muscles come in pairs and run from the back of the orbit to the surface of the sides of the eyeball, beneath the conjunctival membrane. (*See* Figure 2.)

The Sclera and Cornea: The Outer Circle

Three distinct concentric layers of tissue cover the eye. The surface layer (approximately one millimeter thick, roughly the thickness of ten sheets of paper) is made of tough collagen. You see it as both the sclera, a protective coating of collagen and elastic tissue that makes up the white of your eye, and the cornea, a clear, domelike window at the front of the eye. The cornea is the part of the eye on which you would put a contact lens. Light enters your eye through the cornea; the cornea also helps focus light on the retina, the point of convergence of vision at the back of your eye.

Your Eye's Midsection

The middle layer of the eye, called the *uveal tract,* is comprised of the iris, the ciliary body, and the choroid. The *cil-*

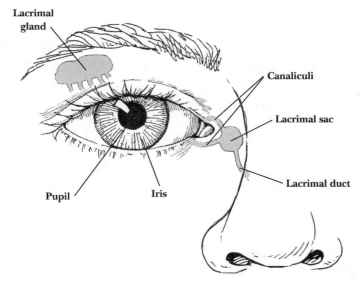

FIGURE 1

The eye: Light enters the eye through the pupil. The colored iris, which is made of muscle fibers, *contracts* or *dilates* (opens or closes) when light is brighter or dimmer. The *lacrimal gland,* located behind the upper lid, produces tears that keep the eye lubricated and clean.

iary body, a structure made up of muscles, blood, and surface cells, produces *aqueous humor,* the waterlike fluid that fills the eye. The middle layer also houses the *ciliary muscles,* which change the shape of the lens to focus the light. The *choroid,* a thin membrane behind the ciliary muscle, is replete with blood vessels; it supplies nutrients to eye tissue, including the rods and cones of the retina, which are specialized light-sensitive cells that respond to color and light.

The Iris and Lens: Light Gatekeepers

The *iris*—the pigmented segment of your eye that denotes

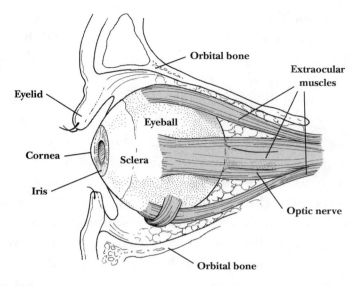

FIGURE 2

Eye anatomy: The eyeball is surrounded by ligaments, fat, and muscles, and rests in a protective, bony socket called the *orbit*. Six extraocular muscles control the eyeball's movement. The *cornea*, a tough, transparent dome that helps focus light, and the *sclera*, the white portion of the eye, protects the interior of the eye. The optic nerve delivers visual information to the brain.

whether you have blue, green, or brown eyes—forms a ring around the *pupil*, a black hole in the iris's center. Essentially a curtain of muscle fibers, the iris controls how much light enters the eye. Like an automatic camera, which adjusts the size of its *aperture* (opening) in response to the available light, the involuntary circular muscles of the iris contract in bright light, making the pupil smaller, and dilate in dim light, making the pupil larger. A good example of the eye's adaptation is the mildly painful change that occurs when you walk into sunlight after sitting for hours in a dark movie theater; or walk into a dark restaurant after being outside on a sunny day. Even the most subtle alterations in light prompt a response from the eye, and the iris muscles are continually working behind the scenes to adjust to the environment.

Just behind the pupil and the iris lies the *crystalline lens,* a flexible, transparent globular body that focuses rays of light onto the *retina,* the thin, light-sensitive layer at the rear of the eye. (*See* Figure 3.) The iris is connected at its outer equator to the ciliary body. The flexible lens behind the iris focuses light rays on the retina with the help of the ciliary muscles in the ciliary body, permitting the lens to alter its shape to allow the eye to focus on objects at varying distances. The ciliary muscles change the shape of the lens by ligaments known as *zonules.* When you look out the window at a tree far away, for instance, the muscles relax and stretch the zonule ligaments, which, in turn, pull on the lens, causing it to flatten and assume a thin contour. However, when you shift your gaze to something close, such as a computer screen, the muscles contract and loosen the zonules, which makes the lens thicker and more curved in the middle. The ability of the lens to focus from far to near is called *accommodation.*

Aqueous Humor

In addition to its focusing function, the surface of the ciliary body of the eye contains cells that produce *aqueous humor,* the watery fluid that provides nutrients to the eye's lens. The aqueous humor is found principally in the space between the iris and the cornea, known as the *anterior chamber.* (See Figure 3.) The fluid flows from the ciliary

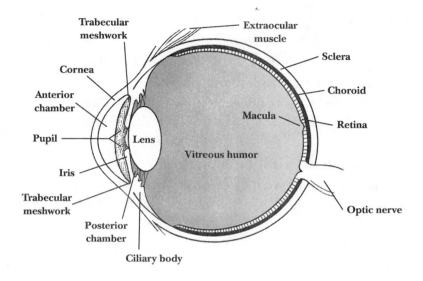

FIGURE 3

Cross-section of the eye: Rays of light pass through the cornea, the anterior chamber, then through the lens, which focuses images. The lens is nourished by the *aqueous humor,* a clear, watery solution that circulates from the posterior chamber into the anterior chamber and helps maintain normal pressure. Light reaches the retina after it passes from the lens through the *vitreous humor,* a clear gel that fills the posterior two-thirds of the eyeball. The retina has light-sensitive cells that capture images, which are then sent to the brain via the optic nerve. At the retina's center is the *macula,* a small region that provides sharp central vision.

body behind the iris into the *posterior chamber*—the area between the iris and the lens. The aqueous humor then goes through the pupil into the anterior chamber, carrying nutrition (and waste products) from the eye into *Schlemm's canal,* a circular drainage system located where the clear cornea, white sclera, and iris meet. In a healthy eye, this circulation constantly drains and resupplies the aqueous humor, maintaining a balance of fluid in the two chambers.

The Vitreous Humor: Your Eye's Support Staff

Behind the lens is the *vitreous humor*, a clear, stable gel, similar to raw egg white, that supports and fills the posterior two-thirds of the eyeball; this gel provides an open pathway for light after it has been focused by the lens.

Your Eye's Innermost Chamber

The posterior part of this middle layer of the eye is the *choroid*, a membrane sandwiched between the sclera and retina in the rear of the eye. The choroid is packed with blood vessels that carry oxygen and other nourishment to the adjacent outer portion of the retina. Taking up nearly three-fourths of the rear inner surface of the eye is the *retina*. Somewhat like the film in a camera, the retina is where images are captured and recorded. It's a mass of unique nerve cells and fibers that relay visual messages to the brain about an object's size, shape, color, and distance. The images are sent as electrical impulses along the optic nerve, which then carries the signal to the brain, where the image is registered.

EYE OPENER

The optic nerve is a bundle of more than one million nerve fibers that carries all visual information from the retina to the brain.

The Retina: Command Central

Within the retina are about 150 million *rods* and 7 million *cones*—specialized cells made up of chemicals that react to different wavelengths of light. Rods, located mainly in the periphery of the retina, don't perceive color but are most sensitive in the dark (where colors are poorly seen). The cones, receptors for color, are responsible for fine detail in the center of vision; they allow us to read the words on a page and recognize a familiar face from across the room. Cones are most active in bright light, which explains why it's hard to detect colors and fine details in the dark. The cones are located primarily in the *macula,* a remarkably small part of the retina that gives us sharp central vision. The best vision—for reading or detail work—comes from the *fovea,* at the center of the macula. The rest of the retina delivers *peripheral* (side) vision, which is less sharply focused.

The Art of Seeing

Your eyesight isn't fully developed at birth; the brain and eyes have to learn to work together in the first months of life. Once sight is well developed—generally by nine or so months of age—the eyes and brain have teamed up to provide virtually instantaneous visual information. Consider what happens when you walk through a parking lot and spot your car. First, you're not actually looking at the car, but at the light reflected off it that enters your eye; there must always be some light present for you to see.

If the image is clear, it means that the light thrown off every surface spot of the car hits your cornea, where it's *refracted,* or bent, inward and is then sent through the aqueous fluid until it reaches the lens. The light rays are then bent further, passed through the vitreous fluid, and projected onto the retina first as a flat, upside-down image. The light is absorbed by the retina and turned into electrical energy, which the optic nerve then conveys to the visual center of the brain as a chemical signal. Data about your car—its size, shape, color, and position—are sent along the optic nerve as *impulses,* a sort of neurologic code that the brain deciphers. The image is actually upside down on the retina but, as part of the learned process of seeing, the brain automatically turns it right side up. (If the image of your car isn't clear, you could have one of several eyesight disorders, from nearsightedness to cataract, many of which are discussed later in this book.)

Although it's possible to see with only one eye, you need *binocular* vision—vision with both eyes—to achieve depth perception. Thus, only with two eyes do you get a complete three-dimensional view of your vehicle because the brain interprets what is seen from two eyes (each with a slightly different perspective) as a single image. Though the flashy car nearby may catch your attention, you can instantly shift your gaze without a thought, because the external muscles are neurologically synchronized to keep the eyes and each eye's image aligned and in focus.

Summary

☛ Although it's just an inch in diameter, the eyeball is a sophisticated system of specialized tissue, nerves, muscles, and cells that work together with the brain to focus light and respond to color. The eyes and brain team up to provide virtually instantaneous visual information. Eyesight is often compared to an autofocus camera, but it's far more complex than that.

☛ Almost like magic, eyesight occurs when the cornea, the thin transparent tissue at the front of the eye, *refracts* (bends) reflected light. It's then focused by the lens and projected onto the *retina,* a layer of specialized cells at the back of the eye that converts light into electrical energy. This electrical energy is then transferred by the optic nerve to the visual center of the brain, where it registers as an image.

☛ Eyes are designed to last a lifetime, although, like the rest of the body, they do change with age.

2

Eye Changes with Age

Just as hair turns gray and skin sags, the eyes, too, undergo a metamorphosis as the years pass. Though many of these changes are part of normal aging, some are not. Abnormal changes associated with aging set the stage for more serious vision problems.

In older eyes, lid muscles weaken, and the skin becomes thinner and more flaccid; this can cause the skin of the upper eyelid to droop somewhat, or the skin of the lower lid to sag. Eyelashes and eyebrows may lose their lushness as they thin considerably. Tear production also drops off as we get older, and the oily film that tears provide to keep the eye surface smooth and clear decreases. This occurs because the lubricating glands in your eyelids and the *conjunctiva,* the transparent membrane that lines the eyelid and covers the front portion of the eye, fail to do their job as well as they once did.

These changes may lead to a buildup of mucus, resulting in stickiness, or drying of the *cornea,* the curved transparent tissue that makes up the front of your eye, irritating your eyes or causing an uncomfortable gritty sensation. You may be able to alleviate some discomfort by regularly applying artificial-tear eye drops, which are sold over the counter.

With age, the conjunctiva also turns thinner, becomes more fragile, and takes on a yellowish tinge from an increase in elastic fibers. The *sclera* (the white of your eye) also yellows, due to a collection of *lipid* (fat) deposits. The exposed conjunctiva between the lids also undergoes degenerative changes, and the cornea, the transparent dome on the eye's surface, may develop an opaque white ring around its periphery called *arcus senilis*.

Lens Changes as Your Eyes Age

As you get older, of course, your eye's lens does, too. In time, it hardens and becomes less elastic, making it more difficult to focus on near objects, a common condition called *presbyopia*. (*See* "Presbyopia," page 122.) Due to these lens changes, you may also find that your night vision grows poorer. These changes usually occur in both eyes simultaneously.

EYE OPENER

You can't ward off presbyopia. Everyone experiences some degree of it as part of aging.

Aging may also cause your eye's crystalline lens to darken, grow opaque, and, in some cases, thicken, resulting in *myopia* (nearsightedness), which means that you have trouble focusing on distant objects—actually a type of early cataract change. Another common type of cataract, the clouding of the lens, usually takes years to develop. The risk of cataract increases with age; you may not notice that you have a cataract until your vision blurs or becomes impaired in your central line of sight. (*See* "Protecting Your Eyes from Cataracts," page 49.)

Over time, the eyes' *anterior* (front) chamber may also become shallower in some susceptible individuals, for example, those who have small eyes, and who are farsighted (have trouble seeing anything close). This farsighted condition increases the risk for blockage of the aqueous humor drainage system by the peripheral iris. As a result of the iris blocking the trabecular meshwork and Schlemm's canal, fluid can back up and lead to increased pressure, which can damage the optic nerve, a serious disease called *closed-angle glaucoma*. If left untreated, closed-angle glaucoma can cause blindness. If treated early by laser, the risk of chronic closed-angle glaucoma can be eliminated. *Open-angle glaucoma* occurs when pressure builds up in the eye not because of the iris blocking the drainage system, but because of a blockage within Schlemm's canal, which is deeper in the eye's drainage pathway. Chronic open-angle glaucoma is often inherited, but is also age-related.

Internal Changes in Older Eyes

As you get older, the *vitreous humor,* the clear gelatinous substance that fills the eyeball, also shows wear and tear, sometimes fragmenting into harmless little clumps of collagen, called *floaters*. (*See* "Floaters," page 138, and "Flashes," page 139.) In many people, the vitreous may separate from the back of the retina, technically called a *posterior vitreous detachment*. A vitreous detachment in and of itself isn't a problem. However, in about one in ten people with a posterior vitreous detachment, a tear in the retina may develop. Flashing lights or a shower of floaters may signal that this type of tear has occurred. These floaters may be composed of retinal cells or blood. In some retinal tears, fluid may collect behind the retina, detaching it from underlying tissue in the same way that water trapped behind wallpaper causes it to peel. Fortunately, if a retinal tear is caught early, before fluid collects, it may be repaired using a laser, with no visual loss. If the retina does detach, it usually requires surgical repair in an operating room. (*See* "Retinal Detachment," page 140.)

Also with age, the *retina*—the innermost layer of the eye, which converts light to electrical energy—thins and grows less sensitive due to cell loss, a decreased blood supply, or degeneration. Especially prone to deterioration is the *macula,* the most sensitive part of the retina; age-related macular degeneration is a serious disease that can steal a person's central vision. (*See* "Protecting Your Sight from Age-Related Macular Degeneration," page 107.)

EYE OPENER

The macula—the central area of the retina—is the most active part of the eye; its light-sensing nerve cells are constantly working to allow you to see fine detail, such as threading a needle or reading newspaper print.

It's estimated that someone in America goes blind every 11 minutes. Although that sounds like a lot, the good news is that, in actuality, many people never develop eye disease and maintain their vision well into old age. In all likelihood, as you grow older, with proper eye care, you will need little more than reading glasses and stronger illumination, such as brighter lights around your house—at kitchen counters, stairways, and favorite reading places. Besides helping you see better, more illumination can help prevent accidents caused by weaker eyesight.

In those who develop age-related eye diseases, however, early treatment can often help stop disease from progressing. The key is proper eye care and timely diagnosis.

Summary

☛ Just as hair turns gray, eyes change as you age. Eyelids weaken and become thinner. The tissues of the eyes become more fragile, and the lens of the eye becomes less elastic. Although many eye changes are part of normal aging, some are not. Abnormal changes associated with aging, such as deterioration of the *macula*, the most sensitive part of the retina, set the stage for more serious vision problems.

☛ Most people never develop eye disease, and will need little more than reading glasses and stronger lighting as they grow older. Still, it's important to see an eye doctor regularly.

☛ Treatment won't reverse an age-related eye disease, such as cataract or glaucoma, but it can often help stop the disease in its tracks and preserve vision.

3

Eye-Care Basics: Getting Your Eyes Examined

Regular, comprehensive eye exams are your best defense against eye disease. Younger people with normal eyes, no particular problems, and no family risk factors don't need frequent exams—every three to five years is sufficient. For people ages forty to sixty-four, without eye diseases or risk factors for disease, the American Academy of Ophthalmology recommends an exam every two to four years. If you're sixty-five or older, you should schedule an exam with an *ophthalmologist,* a medical doctor who specializes in treating the eyes, every one to two years—even if you have no noticeable symptoms.

Those who are at greater risk for specific eye conditions because of age, family history, or other risk factors should schedule certain exams more frequently. If you're not sure whether you're at increased risk for eye disease, talk to your eye doctor. In general, you're at higher risk for eye disease if you're middle-aged or older; if you have diabetes or another disease in which eyesight may be affected; if you have a family history of eye disease; and-or have had a past eye injury.

A thorough eye exam involves a series of evaluations, some done in the dark, some in the light, and some with special instruments. If you've never had a comprehensive eye exam, now's the time. Make an appointment with your eye doctor today.

WHEN TO SEE AN EYE DOCTOR

Have your eyes examined every two to four years by an optometrist or ophthalmologist if you're between forty and sixty-four, and every one to two years by an ophthalmologist after age sixty-five, even if you aren't experiencing any discomfort or eye problems. (Some potentially serious eye diseases are symptomless, especially in their early, most treatable stages.) You should also be sure to see an ophthalmologist if you experience any of the following symptoms or problems, even if you were seen by an eye doctor recently:

- bulging of the eyes
- change in the color of the iris
- crossed eyes
- dark spot in the center of your field of vision
- difficulty focusing on near or distant objects
- double vision
- dry eyes with itching or burning
- excess discharge or tearing

- eye pain
- floaters or flashes
- *haloes* (colored circles around lights)
- hazy or blurred vision
- loss of peripheral vision
- redness of or around the eye
- spots in your field of vision
- straight lines appear wavy or crooked
- sudden loss of vision
- trouble adjusting to dark rooms
- unusual sensitivity to light or glare
- veil, blocking vision

Reviewing Your Health History

Before the exam, the physician will ask about your current and past health, including your general well-being, childhood diseases, allergies, and personal and family history of medical problems. Be sure to mention any diseases you have, drug allergies, and whether you've had any eye injuries, infections, or operations. These details, especially your family history, are important in assessing your risk of eye disease. Some eye disorders are associated with heredity, and some with disease. Diabetes, for example, can affect vision, and always deserves careful attention.

The doctor will also ask if you wear glasses or contact lenses, how you care for them, and when you wear them. In a routine exam, the eye doctor will inquire about any changes in your general health, over-the-counter and pre-scription medicines you're taking, and any new vision complaints since your last exam.

QUESTIONS TO ASK YOUR EYE DOCTOR

At your eye appointment, it's important to become informed, so that you and your doctor can work together to protect and maintain your eye health. If your doctor detects an eye problem, here are some key questions you may want to ask to help you best understand your disease or disorder and treatment.

1. What kinds of diagnostic tests do I need? Do I need to do anything special to prepare for them?
2. What is my diagnosis?
3. What's the treatment for my condition?
4. When will treatment start and how long will it last?
5. Are there any side effects of treatment that I should be aware of?
6. Are there foods, drugs, or activities I should avoid while I'm undergoing this treatment?
7. How may this condition affect my vision now and in the future?
8. Are there any particular symptoms I should watch for?
9. What should I do if these symptoms occur?
10. Will changing my diet, exercise, or other lifestyle habits help improve my condition?

To fully understand your condition and make decisions about your own health care, take notes or get a friend or family member to take notes for you during your eye appointment. Eye diseases can be complicated and confusing. If necessary, consider bringing a tape recorder with you to record your office visit, so that you can jot down important information about your condition and your doctor's advice later. (As a courtesy, be sure to ask your doctor for permission to record your conversation.) You might also consider doing your own research about your condition. (The "Resources" section, page 229, is a good place to start.) By being more informed, you will be able to communicate better with your eye doctor and feel more in control of the situation.

EYE PROFESSIONALS

If you've ever been confused about whether you need to see an ophthalmologist, optometrist, or optician, you're not alone; the names of the specialists sound similar. However, each plays a distinct role in eye care. Because the training and experience of each specialist varies, it's important to seek the services of the appropriate provider for your eye-care needs.

Ophthalmologists:

An *ophthalmologist* is a physician—either a doctor of medicine (M.D.) or doctor of osteopathy (D.O.)—who specializes in the medical and surgical care of the eyes and visual system, as well as in the prevention of eye disease. To become a licensed ophthalmologist, a doctor must have completed four or more years of medical school, one year of internship, and three or more years of specialized medical, surgical, and refractive training. Ophthalmologists are qualified to diagnose and treat (medically and surgically) all diseases, disorders, and injuries of the eyes and visual system. In addition, they may provide more basic eye care, including prescribing eyeglasses and contact lenses.

Optometrists:

Optometrists are doctors of optometry and are health-service providers who deal with vision problems. They must have completed a four-year course at an accredited college of optometry, but don't attend medical school and aren't trained to perform surgery. Optometrists are state licensed to examine the eyes, determine the presence of vision problems (including eye diseases), recommend eye exercises, and prescribe eyeglasses and contact lenses. In many states, optometrists are permitted to treat certain eye conditions with topical or therapeutic drugs. Normally, if an optometrist diagnoses a patient with a serious eye disorder, he or she will refer that patient to an ophthalmologist for further treatment.

Opticians:

An optician is a technician who makes, fits, and delivers eyeglasses, contact lenses, or other optical devices after they've been prescribed by an ophthalmologist or optometrist.

Testing Your Vision

After reviewing your personal and family medical history, your doctor is likely to have you read from the *Snellen chart*, the familiar chart with the rows of letters and numbers that diminish in size. By using this chart, the doctor can test your visual acuity—the sharpness of your central vision. If you wear corrective lenses, your vision will be tested with your current prescription. The doctor will also look at your glasses through a device called a *lensometer* to ascertain your exact prescription. You will be scored according to how well you see compared to someone with normal vision. For instance, if you have normal 20/20 vision, that means you can see at a distance of twenty feet what an individual with standard vision sees at twenty feet. However, if your vision is 20/40, you see at a distance of twenty feet what a person with normal vision would be able to see at forty feet; in other words, you need to stand closer to the object to see it as clearly. The general rule: the higher the second number, the worse your vision. This rule applies to everyone, no matter if you're near- or farsighted.

If the Snellen test indicates a need for corrective lenses or a prescription adjustment, the doctor will measure your eye's *refraction,* or focusing error, using instruments that contain a combination of different strengths of corrective lenses. (*See* Figure 4.) To confirm that reading, you will be tested subjectively, using a variety of lenses, to ascertain which one gives you the best sight.

How well you see peripherally will also be evaluated; typically, you'll be asked to cover one eye and fix the other eye on a point straight ahead. The ophthalmologist will shift an object, such as a pen, back and forth at the outer edges of your visual field and ask you to note when you see it moving. If followup is necessary, specialized equipment can map the extent of your peripheral vision.

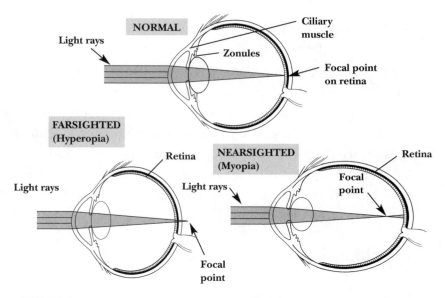

FIGURE 4

Refractive errors: When the eye sees normally, light focuses directly on the retina, producing a sharp image. In a farsighted person, light rays reach the retina before they can be focused. This happens either because the eyeball is too short from front to back, or the lens and cornea have diminished refractive power. Thus, it is easier to see distant objects more clearly than those that are close. In a nearsighted person, light rays focus in front of the retina due to either an elongated eyeball, or an overpowered lens or cornea. Close objects can be seen clearly, but those at a distance are blurred.

EYE OPENER

As the years go by, you may notice that you may need more light to see, and that it's more difficult to tell the difference between some colors, such as shades of blue and green. Don't worry. These are natural vision changes associated with eyes "of a certain age."

Examining the External Eye

During your eye exam, your eye doctor will also examine the outer eye—the lids, lashes, and orbit—to look for signs of any underlying problems, such as infections, styes, cysts, tumors, or lid-muscle weaknesses. The physician will study your eyeball's appearance (including the *sclera,* the white of your eye and *conjunctiva,* the thin membrane covering your eye), and the doctor will note whether your pupil reacts normally to light.

Checking Eye Coordination

Your doctor will also check the coordination of the six muscles in each of your eyes; this is an important part of the exam. Tests may vary but, essentially, the physician wants to ensure your eyes function properly together. Normally, the brain coordinates the eyes by aligning the images into a single three-dimensional picture. To test the alignment of your eyes, the doctor will tell you to focus on some target and alternately cover and uncover each eye with a black plastic spoon. This interrupts the fusion of the eyes and can reveal a tendency for either eye to drift. In a separate test, the doctor will have you follow a penlight with your gaze to determine whether your range of motion is normal, and whether your eyes move in harmony.

Examining the Internal Eye

To check the health of the tissue in the front third of each eye and the ability of the lens to focus, the doctor will use *biomicroscopy,* often called "the slit-lamp exam." During this test, the doctor will use a *slit lamp,* a diagnostic tool with a powerful microscope and a narrow slit of light, to explore different levels of the transparent tissue and the inner workings of the eye.

As you keep your head steady on a chin rest, beams of light are projected onto and into the eye. The instrument's use of narrow light beams and high magnification provides an important cross-sectional picture of eye tissue. The slit lamp thus affords a special view of the cornea, your eye's anterior chamber, the lens, and vitreous humor.

The doctor will check for many things, including degeneration of the cornea, the presence of foreign particles in the cornea, inflammation within the anterior chamber, cataract, tumors, or abnormal blood vessels in the iris. The ophthalmologist can rule out hundreds of conditions during the internal eye examination with the slit-lamp exam.

EYE OPENER

Your eyes are a reflection of your overall health. During an eye exam, diabetes, high blood pressure, and, sometimes, even AIDS, can be detected. With each of these conditions, the sooner they're detected, the better your chances are for being treated successfully.

NEARSIGHTED? FARSIGHTED?

When the eye sees normally, light focuses directly on the retina, producing a clear image. In some people, however, the optics are faulty, and images appear blurred, because the eye focuses the image either in front of or behind the retina. (See Figure 4.) Near- and farsightedness aren't eye diseases, but common problems known as *refractive errors of the eye,* which can be corrected with eyeglasses, contact lenses, or, more recently, by laser surgery.

Myopia (nearsightedness):

A nearsighted person has difficulty seeing objects at a distance, such as street signs, because the light rays converge and focus before reaching the retina. This is usually due to an elongated eyeball (which requires light rays to travel a greater distance than a normal eye does) or a lens or cornea that is too strong, bending the light rays, so that they focus before getting to the retina.

Myopia is often hereditary. It generally starts in the elementary-school years and may progress into the late twenties or early thirties. Glasses or contacts with concave lenses that are thick on the edges and thinner in the middle are necessary to focus the image on the retina. Laser surgery, including the newest form of refractive surgery, called *LASIK* surgery, is being used increasingly to correct myopia and reduce or eliminate the need for glasses. (For more information on LASIK surgery, *see* page 73.)

Hyperopia (farsightedness):

People with this defect see objects better at a distance than up close. In this case, the eyeball is usually too short, and light rays reach the retina before they are focused. Farsightedness can also be caused by weaknesses in the refractive power of the lens and cornea. Farsighted children and young adults often don't experience blurred vision with farsightedness because their eyes can compensate for it. The muscles of their eyes make the lens rounder, which allows the image to focus on the retina and creates a clear image. This accommodation occurs involuntarily. If you're farsighted, you may develop headaches and eyestrain if the condition isn't corrected with eyeglasses or contact lenses.

While farsightedness may go unnoticed for years, the eye's corrective ability diminishes with age, and a farsighted person may need glasses by midlife. Convex lenses with thick centers and thin edges greatly improve close vision. In addition, laser surgery may be used to correct some degrees of hyperopia.

Astigmatism:

In this condition, irregularities in the curvature of the surface of the *cornea,* the transparent dome on the front surface of the eye, cause distorted vision. Light rays don't meet at a single point, so images may focus at two different places along the visual axis. For some people, vertical lines appear blurry; for others, horizontal or diagonal lines may look out of focus. Perhaps the problem can best be explained this way: If a person bends a flexible flat mirror and looks into it, the face is distorted by the astigmatic surface of the mirror. Glasses that have a similar degree of curvature, but in the opposite direction, correct the distorted image.

Astigmatism develops early and is usually well established after the first few years of life. The defect often occurs together with nearsightedness or farsightedness, and can be corrected with curved lenses.

Testing Pupil Dilation

The ophthalmologist may use drops of a dilating drug to enlarge the pupils. This procedure allows the doctor to better examine the eye's interior. The effect of the drops, however, takes time to wear off, so you may experience light sensitivity and difficulty focusing on close tasks for several hours if reversal drops aren't used. If your pupils are dilated, you may be advised to wear sunglasses outside and to avoid driving and wearing contact lenses until your vision returns to normal.

Measuring Eye Pressure (*Tonometry*)

During your eye exam, you can also expect your doctor to measure the internal pressure in your eyes to detect possible signs of glaucoma and optic-nerve damage. During this painless test, each eye is numbed with anesthetic drops. The doctor then touches the cornea with an instrument called an *applanation tonometer,* to measure the eye's resistance to flattening the surface of the cornea to the surface of the tonometer. In an alternative—but less accurate—procedure, a puff of air is blown against the eye to determine the force it takes to flatten the cornea. Anyone at risk for glaucoma, including everyone over age forty or anyone who has a borderline result with the puff-of-air test, should insist on also being tested with the more accurate applanation tonometer. (For more information on glaucoma, *see* page 77.)

Viewing the Retina and Optic Nerve

Finally, the doctor will use a hand-held *ophthalmoscope,* an instrument with focusing lenses and a light source or the slit lamp, to look more deeply into your eye. The ophthalmoscope has an angled mirror, various lenses, and a light source. With it, the doctor can see the *vitreous humor* (fluid in the eye), the retina, the macula, the head of the optic nerve and the surrounding blood vessels, the retinal veins, and arteries.

In special circumstances, the doctor will use different lenses to view the far periphery of the retina. The light source may be mounted on the doctor's head or at the slit lamp.

If you think your eyes are too sensitive or if you're afraid of an eye exam because you think it may be painful, rest assured. An eye exam isn't anything to be frightened of, especially now that you're informed and know what to expect. Everything is painless!

Summary

☛ Regular eye exams are the best defense against age-related eye disease. People ages forty to sixty-four without eye diseases or risk factors for disease should have an exam every two to four years. Those sixty-five or older should schedule an exam with an *ophthalmologist,* a medical doctor who specializes in treating the eyes, every one to two years—even if they have no noticeable symptoms. More frequent visits may be needed if there's a family history of eye disease or another condition that increases the risk for eye disease.

☞ A thorough eye exam involves a battery of tests that examines the inner and external workings of the eye to check for infections and signs of macular degeneration, glaucoma, cataracts, and other problems. An eye exam is a painless procedure, so there's no need to worry about discomfort.

☞ If an eye problem is diagnosed, it's important to understand diagnosis and treatment by asking your doctor specific questions, such as any subsequent diagnostic tests you may need to confirm the initial diagnosis. Preserving vision is a working partnership between the patient and the eye doctor. Don't be afraid to ask the doctor to clarify anything you don't understand.

4

Protecting Your Eyes from Cataracts

Think of how a pane of glass appears when it's dirty— that's how the interior of the eye's crystalline lens looks when a cataract develops. In a normal eye, light passes through the clear lens and is focused on the *retina,* the eye's light-sensitive layer that works with the optic nerve to send visual signals to the brain where they become an image. In an eye with a cataract, however, the lens becomes foggy and the opacity either prevents light from reaching the retina or distorts the light rays, both of which may cause a disabling loss of vision.

According to the National Eye Institute, cataract occurs in about half of all Americans age sixty-five and over. Each year, approximately 1.5 million cataract surgeries are performed in the United States, making it one of the most successful and commonly performed operations in the country. Between the ages of fifty-two and sixty-four, you have a

50 percent chance of having a cataract but, according to the American Academy of Ophthalmology, you probably won't experience any problems until about age sixty-five. Despite surgical advances, cataract remains the leading preventable cause of blindness in the world today, but that's mainly due to limited access to health care in less-developed countries.

EYE OPENER

In the United States, age-related cataracts cost $5 billion a year to extract and otherwise treat, the largest single item on Medicare expenditures.

What Causes Cataracts?

Misconceptions abound when it comes to cataracts. Contrary to popular belief, cataracts aren't caused by cancer or a film blanketing the eye. It's not related to overuse of the eyes, and doesn't spread from one eye to the other—although the condition may develop in both eyes.

Natural aging and the accompanying changes in the chemical composition of the lens are the most common causes of cataracts. Many cataracts develop as an exaggeration of normal aging *sclerosis,* in which the lens becomes less resilient, less transparent and often thicker. According to clinical studies, more than 40 percent of people in their fifties to early sixties already have some sclerosis in their lenses. Fibers in the lens become compressed, and the lens turns more rigid. The lens is mostly made of protein and water, arranged in a precise way to keep the lens clear, and let light pass through. However, if these proteins *coagulate*, or clump together, creating tiny specks or wheellike spokes in the periphery of the lens, clarity fades. Other cataracts may develop at the center of the lens, causing nearsighted-ness, before opacity and distortion. In later stages of cataract development, the milkiness becomes denser and occurs in the center, making it truly difficult to see. The change in the lens is similar to what happens when an egg white is boiled: It goes from clear to opaque.

.

EYE OPENER

During middle age, cataracts are typically small, and most don't affect vision.

Although age is the factor most likely to cause cataracts, heredity, eye injuries, some medications (par-ticularly corticosteroids), and certain health problems, such as diabetes, may cause cataracts as well. Several studies have linked cataracts with alcohol consumption and smoking. Even if you have smoked for many years, quitting now will help you avoid cataract in the future. (See "There Has Never Been a Better Time to Stop Smoking," page 171.) Long-term exposure to high lev-els of ultraviolet-A (UVA) and ultraviolet-B (UVB) rays from the sun is another hazard, as studies have found a greater prevalence of cataract in people who live in areas with considerable sunlight. An important 1988 study found high percentages of cataracts and lens opacities among Maryland fishermen who worked outdoors all their lives.

On rare occasions, a baby may be born with cataracts—the consequence of some problem that affected the fetus during pregnancy, such as the mother's exposure to German measles during the first trimester. Cataract may also be inherited from either the father or mother.

Symptoms of Cataracts

At first, cataracts affect vision only slightly. You may notice that your vision is a little blurred, like looking through a filmy piece of glass. The disorder is painless and progresses slowly. As the cataract gets bigger or "ripens," vision usually becomes more blurry or dim, like trying to see through a waterfall, and glare from lights and the sun becomes especially distressing. You may also experience double vision, as well as a distorted image. In the early stages, the eye may even become more nearsighted because, the denser the lens, the greater its refracting power. Your night vision is also apt to worsen, and colors may appear less vivid. You may also find it difficult to read and do other normal tasks.

Because most cataracts develop slowly, you may not understand what's wrong, until the decline in your visual acuity forces you to seek frequent changes in your eyeglass or contact lens prescription. These efforts are usually fruitless, however, because corrective lenses can't reverse the opacity of cataract.

CATARACT: WHAT TO WATCH FOR

Watch out for any of these symptoms in one or both eyes. Any may indicate that a cataract is developing:

- blurry, cloudy, or dim vision
- glare from bright lights, such as lamps or bright sunlight
- double or multiple vision
- distorted images
- increasing nearsightedness
- declining night vision
- frequent changes in your eyeglass or contact lens prescription

Diagnosing Cataracts

Anyone who experiences blurring or eye discomfort should visit an ophthalmologist immediately for a full examination, because cataract is only one of several important diseases that affect vision. (*See* "When to See an Eye Doctor," page 35.) During the exam, the doctor will test the sharpness of your vision with the Snellen chart (see page 39) and probably dilate your pupils with eye drops to see more of the lens and the back of your eye—the retina and the optic nerve—to look for other eye problems. By examining the interior of your eye with a slit lamp, your physician can assess whether a cataract has formed and just how extensive the cloudy patches are. Your doctor will also perform additional examinations to rule out the possibility of other eye disorders, such as glaucoma or retinal detachment.

EYE OPENER

Can Obesity Cause Cataracts?

As you grow older, maintaining a healthy weight is especially important to reduce your risk of certain diseases, including cataract. A recent study that followed over 17,000 apparently healthy male physicians for an average of fourteen years found that those who qualified as obese had a 25 percent greater chance of developing cataract than did men who weren't obese. However, few experts believe that weight itself causes cataracts. Rather, obesity increases the risk of diabetes, which, in turn, increases the risk of cataracts.

Treating Cataracts

Cataract surgery—surgically removing cataracts and replacing them with a substitute lens—is the only effective cure; there are no drugs, eye drops, diets, exercises, or corrective lenses proven to cure or reverse the problem.

When cataract is the only disease present, surgery is usually successful. (*See* Figure 5.) However, a diagnosis of cataract doesn't mean immediate surgery; in a minority of cataract cases, the lens will thicken, causing nearsightedness, rather than becoming opaque. If your vision is only slightly blurry and it isn't interfering with your lifestyle and the things you enjoy doing, you may wish to delay or avoid cataract surgery, in which case, any of these tactics may help compensate for your vision problems:

☞ **New eyeglasses:** Ask your eye doctor about adjusting your eyeglass prescription for distance or stronger bifocals to help you see better. You might also try magnifying lenses for close work. For more information, see "Living with Low Vision," page 147.

☞ **Reducing glare:** Improve lighting at home by using stronger lighting for close work. Position lighting directly on reading material rather than having it shine over your shoulder, and use lamp shades and frosted light bulbs to reduce glare. You might also ask your ophthalmologist about yellow-tinted lenses, which also tend to keep glare to a minimum.

☞ **Eyedrops:** With certain types of cataracts, medications that dilate your pupils allow more light to be transmitted. For more information, speak to your eye doctor.

Also, ask your eye doctor about what you can do to protect and prolong your vision in lieu of cataract surgery. Your eye doctor may have suggestions based on your particular manifestation of the disease. Indeed, many people

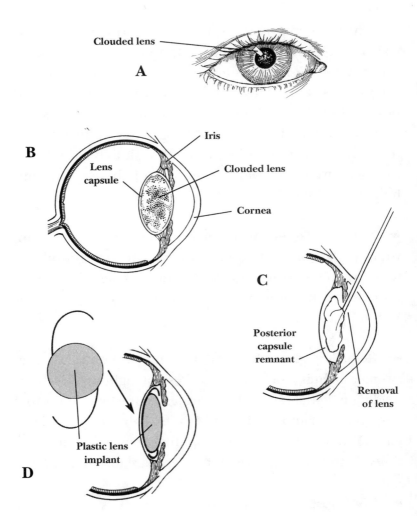

FIGURE 5

Removing a cataract: Half of all people between ages sixty- five and seventy-four and about 70 percent of those who are older develop cataract. Exposure to sunlight, natural aging, and the accompanying changes in the chemical composition of the lens, cause it to lose its transparency and become clouded (A, B). An opaque lens still transmits light so, although visual acuity may be lost, cataract rarely results in total blindness. In phacoemulsification and extracapsular surgery (C), the clouded lens and front part of its capsule are removed. The posterior capsule remains and provides support for an artificial lens (D).

may successfully delay cataract surgery for several years, while others may never need it.

EYE OPENER

According to the American Academy of Ophthalmology, cataract surgery, an elective procedure, is covered by Medicare.

Are You Ready for Cataract Surgery?

When a new prescription and glare-reduction tactics don't work to enhance your vision, you may be a candidate for cataract surgery. In general, it may be time for surgery when your cataract is affecting your day-to-day life. That is, it's time to consider cataract extraction if, because of your vision, you don't feel confident when you drive, you can't do your best work, you can't read comfortably, you're afraid you'll trip and fall, and/or you don't see very well most of the time, even with your glasses.

EYE OPENER

A cataract needs to be removed only when vision loss interferes with your everyday activities or causes concern about your safety, such as when you're driving or maneuvering stairs.

Those who rely on their eyes for detail work, such as architects, dentists, and editors, are likely to require surgery sooner than others are. Discuss your situation with your ophthalmologist, and together make the decision regarding surgery. Most ophthalmologists are trained to perform cataract surgery, or will supply a referral. You may also want to ask around to find an experienced surgeon to guide you through the preparatory, operative, and postoperative stages.

If your doctor determines that you have cataracts in both eyes, she may recommend operating first on the eye with the denser cataract (and poorer vision). Assuming the surgery is successful and your vision is substantially improved, you may not need to have the second cataract removed. However, most patients note significant benefits from also having the second cataract removed, and will frequently choose the second surgery once the healing and vision is stable in the first eye. Again, the decision to operate on your second eye, as well as the decision to operate at all, should be made with your ophthalmologist.

Like all surgery, cataract surgery isn't without risks. Problems after surgery, though rare, may include infection, bleeding, pain, redness and swelling, retinal detachment, light flashes, and even permanent loss of vision.

Cataract Surgery When You See Okay

There are some situations in which your doctor may recommend cataract surgery even if your vision isn't severely impaired. For example, when other eye conditions, such as retinal holes or retinal detachment are present, the doctor may recommend cataract extraction because the cataract gets in the way of properly examining and managing those other problems. Whatever the situation, you and your doctor should discuss the rationale for the operation as well as the benefits and risks. You're in the best position to know how much visual impairment you're experiencing, and to determine how much of it is interfering with your safety and daily activities. Unlike other ocular diseases, whereby only the doctor can tell what measures are necessary, with uncomplicated cataracts, the ophthalmologist's role is to help patients reach their own decisions about surgery.

Removing the Cataract

Years ago, cataract surgery was an inpatient procedure requiring general anesthesia and up to a week's stay in the hospital. Surgeons made an incision about a half-inch long, through which they removed the clouded lens and replaced it with thick glasses or, later, an artificial lens. Today, this commonplace operation is often performed under local anesthesia with an operating microscope on an outpatient basis in less than thirty minutes. Although it isn't risk free, cataract surgery is considered one of the safest surgeries in the United States. To remove a cataract, the surgeon makes a very small incision in the eye, about three-sixteenths of an inch. Unlike some other eye surgeries, cataract surgery doesn't employ the use of lasers except, in some cases, for followup procedures, such as when the *lens capsule*, which houses the lens, turns cloudy.

There are two basic types of cataract surgery: extracapsular and intracapsular.

☞ **Extracapsular surgery:** An incision of about three-eighths of an inch is made under the upper lid, where the sclera and cornea join. After making the incision, the surgeon opens the lens capsule, which houses the lens, and removes the harder, central portion of the lens, usually in one piece. The softer part of the lens is then vacuumed out with a suction instrument. The lens capsule is left undisturbed, providing support for a lens implant, a plastic lens which will now focus light onto the retina, and reduce the incidence of complications with the retina. The surgeon removes only the clouded lens, then stitches the incision. (The stitches are buried and rarely need to be removed. In time, they simply disintegrate.) This technique is typically used for very dense or hard cataracts, and in other special circumstances. Because of the size of the incision, small though it is, healing may take a few weeks.

☞ **Phacoemulsification:** The newest type of extraocular cataract surgery, this is the most common way cataracts are removed today. The doctor makes a tiny incision—only about one-eighth of an inch long—on the side of the cornea. Then, with an ultrasonic probe, high-frequency ultrasound (sound waves) are used to break up the cataract so it can be suctioned out through a tiny, needlelike tube. (See Figure 5.) This method has become widespread because the incision is so small that it often needs no stitches. The natural pressure within the eye simply holds the incision tightly closed, leaving a wound that heals rapidly.

Like general extracapsular surgery, the clouded lens will be replaced with a clear plastic artificial intraocular lens. In this case, an innovative folding lens, made of silicone or acrylic, has been developed specifically for phacoemulsification. The lens is smaller than a dime and folded like a taco to fit into place inside the lens capsule, where it will open fully. However, the surgeon may decide to use a rigid lens with phacoemulsification; in which case, the surgeon will enlarge the incision to insert the implant. Depending on the length of the incision, a stitch or two may be necessary.

Phacoemulsification offers good long-term results and is successful without any complications in 97 to 98 percent of all cases, when done by an experienced surgeon. The main difference between general extracapsular surgery and phacoemulsification is that with "phaco," most patients can resume their normal routine sooner since the incision is one-third the size of that produced in general extracapsular surgery. Overall, either procedure restores vision to 20/40 or better in more than 90 percent of all cases. More than 95 percent of people with intraocular lenses find their vision restored to what it was before the cataract developed. Still, after cataract surgery, you may need to wear glasses for reading or distance vision, especially if you have astigmatism.

☛ **Intracapsular surgery:** In this procedure, which is rare today, the entire cataract (lens plus capsule) is removed. Intracapsular surgery is generally reserved for dislocated cataracts due either to injury or an accompanying disease. In this type of surgery, as in extracapsular surgery, plastic lens implants that are permanently fixed inside the eye to replace the natural lens after cataract extraction may be used. Some people, however, can't have an intraocular lens implanted due to problems during surgery or another eye disease. For these people, a soft contact lens or glasses with powerful magnification may be better options.

THE ARTIFICIAL LENS

More than 99 percent of patients who undergo cataract surgery have an intraocular, or plastic artificial lens permanently implanted in the lens capsule to reduce the incidence of complications with the retina. Once the natural lens is removed, the eye becomes extremely farsighted and loses its ability to focus. In the past, to restore this power, people had to wear ungainly magnifying glasses that often provided a distorted view of the world. These glasses are seldom used today. People who had cataract surgery before implants were available, and those with eye disease that make them poor candidates for a synthetic lens, are often fitted with contact lenses, an excellent visual aid.

An intraocular lens replaces the eye's natural lens; most people who receive an intraocular lens see more clearly afterward. Most often, the intraocular lens is placed directly behind the iris. In rarer cases, it's placed in front of the iris.

An intraocular lens requires no care and becomes a permanent part of your eye. It's corrected to meet your eye's specific needs. You won't see or feel it.

Unlike your natural lens, an intraocular lens can't change shape to focus at varying distances. As a result, the intraocular lens is usually calculated for distance vision, so you can see well enough to move about without glasses. With this in mind, you may still need to wear glasses, especially to read. Glasses are usually fitted about a month after surgery.

EYE OPENER

Most often, the lens implant that replaces the clouded lens will be a posterior chamber lens; that is, it's slipped in behind the iris, within the capsule of the cataract. When it's inserted in front of the iris, as might occur when the capsule is faulty, it's called an anterior chamber lens. In either case, tiny plastic loops hold the lens implant in place.

When an Artificial Lens Isn't an Option

For the less than 1 percent of cataract patients who can't tolerate intraocular lenses due to severe eye inflammation or an accompanying disease, such as rheumatoid arthritis, the ophthalmologist will remove the lens but not substitute anything for it. Instead, the doctor will prescribe contact lenses or cataract eyeglasses to correct postoperative vision. Cataract glasses affect vision differently from regular eyeglasses. Their powerful magnification may make it more difficult to judge distance, and may distort vision. Until one has adjusted to these changes, extra care must be taken when driving and doing other potentially dangerous activities.

THE EVOLUTION OF CATARACT SURGERY

For centuries, cataracts have stolen sight from millions of people. One of the first means of cataract removal was practiced nearly three-thousand years ago in India, and also in the region around the Mediterranean Sea. This early method, called couching, displaced the cataract, moving it out of the line of sight into the vitreous humor, by a sharp blow to the eye. Although couching often resulted in glaucoma and blindness, it was commonly practiced in some countries until recently; even today, couching is done in some areas of the world. Scientists eventually learned more about the eye and the formation of cataracts. Surgeons first tried intracapsular extraction in the late nineteenth century, though it wasn't until the 1930s and 1940s that this technique was refined and came into common use.

One successful method that became popular in the 1960s was cryo-intracapsular extraction, in which the doctor applied a freezing probe to the whole lens to make it easier to remove. Extracapsular surgery was performed with and without sutures as early as fifty years ago. However, the recuperation for both early intra- and extraocular surgery was lengthy; patients were laid up for weeks, their heads supported with pillows and sandbags to give the wound time to heal. With the advent of microsurgery and more precise instruments, there was a return to extracapsular extraction. The development of smaller and finer needles and suture material further advanced cataract surgery, allowing surgeons to close wounds with less risk.

A British ophthalmologist, Harold Ridley, implanted the first intraocular lens in 1949. The operation grew out of his observation during World War II, when a fighter pilot was unharmed when plastic from his plane's shattered windshield lodged in his eye. That early artificial lens was crude and led to numerous complications. Today, however, technology is so advanced that nearly everyone receives an intraocular lens after cataract surgery. Technology today even offers, in selected cases, bifocal and multifocal implants.

Preparing for Cataract Surgery

Before cataract surgery, the ophthalmologist will measure the curvature of your cornea, and the size and shape of your eye, to calculate the power and type of the intraocular implant that will be placed in your eye during surgery, if appropriate. Your doctor or clinician will perform a general medical exam, and may take photographs of your eye. To assess the general state of your health, your eye doctor may also do blood tests and an electrocardiogram to check your heart. For several days, you may be advised to avoid aspirin and other drugs that have an anticoagulant effect, especially if the surgery involves the larger incisions. Cataract surgery may also be performed safely on patients who, for medical reasons, must take aspirin or anticoagulants. If you're on medication, be sure to ask your doctor if you should continue.

You'll probably be advised to avoid eating or drinking anything the night and morning before surgery. Once you arrive at the hospital or outpatient clinic, you may be given medication to put you at ease. Next, the hospital staff will clean the area around your eye, and cover your head with sterile sheets so that only the eye is exposed. An anesthesiologist or registered anesthetic assistant may insert a catheter in your arm to deliver intravenous medicines, if needed. Heart monitors and fresh air or oxygen are commonly used during surgery. Topical eye drops are generally administered to dilate the pupil, and partially numb the eye. The operation may be done under local, or rarely, under general anesthesia; a local anesthetic is preferred, particularly for older people, because there's a reduced risk of complications and a faster recovery following surgery.

The anesthesiologist administers local anesthesia via an injection around the eye to keep the eye from moving. In some cases, anesthesia may include only drops and mild intravenous sedation. The entire procedure usually lasts about thirty minutes, during which you may see light, hear noises, and be aware of the presence of the surgical team. During surgery, you won't experience any pain. Most people can't see formed images and often can't tell whether their eye is open or closed.

What to Expect After Surgery

Once the operation is completed, the surgeon may place a bandage or shield over the affected eye, which may be removed later that day. The doctor will prescribe a course of antibiotics and anti-inflammatory drops that should be started soon after the surgery. Be sure to use them as prescribed. You will usually be discharged after you rest for a while in the recovery area, but you will need someone to accompany you home. Most people who undergo cataract surgery go home the same day. In rare cases, when a complication arises or a patient has some other mitigating health problem, an overnight stay in the hospital may be necessary.

There are few limitations after cataract removal. Once at home, use antibiotics and cortisone drops or ointment to prevent infection and reduce inflammation. Because of the eye's postoperative sensitivity, avoid rubbing or touching your eye, and guard against any sudden movement that could jar your head. You will need to wear a protective metal eye shield for a few days or weeks when sleeping to avoid accidentally rubbing your eye. Your doctor or health professional will show you how to clean your eyelids, which may become crusted from discharge. Most people will need to wear medium-density sunglasses (*see* "Invest in the Right Sunglasses," page 175) when outdoors to screen out glare, even though most implants have ultraviolet blockers.

Make sure you understand all of your doctor's postoperative care instructions. It's important to follow these directions carefully to help ensure a full and rapid recovery. Discuss any questions you have with your physician.

When you get home, try not to bend or lift heavy objects, both of which increase pressure in the eye. You can walk, climb stairs, and do light household chores, although it's a good idea to take it easy. Most people can resume normal activities within a few days. Check with your doctor, however, before doing anything strenuous.

Vision usually improves immediately following cataract surgery. However, in some cases, vision may recover more slowly, taking several days or even a few weeks to return to normal. This doesn't indicate any complication or failure of the surgery. Ask your doctor what to expect, and when you can resume all normal activities, including driving, again. Wear sunglasses and/or your eye shield as your doctor recommends.

Itching, sticky eyelids, sensitivity to light, and mild tearing are perfectly normal after surgery, but severe pain and sudden change in vision are unusual. Report either to your physician immediately. Patients who suffer minor discomfort can take a nonaspirin painkiller for relief every four to six hours (aspirin can cause bleeding). Within a day or two, any discomfort should subside on its own.

During the healing process, you may be surprised by changes in color. The clouded lens, which commonly filters out some colors, has been removed and replaced with an intraocular implant, thus, colors may appear more luminous or seem to cast a bluish glow. Spending time in bright sunlight may give objects a reddish afterimage when you come indoors. Within a few weeks of cataract surgery, these perceptions of brightness and abnormal color should go away. Reading and watching television are permitted almost immediately. The ophthalmologist will schedule several postoperative visits: the day after surgery, after about a week, at three to five weeks, and then, usually, two to three months later. The doctor will periodically examine your eye and its visual acuity and measure eye pressure. Corrections for eyeglasses will probably not be prescribed for three to six weeks following surgery.

Possible Complications

More than 98 percent of patients have improved vision after cataract surgery, assuming no other limiting eye disease, and most have an uneventful recuperation. Complications, mild or severe, are extremely rare, but need immediate medical attention. Eye infections after cataract surgery are very rare, occurring once in several thousand operations. However, if an infection develops inside the eye, vision—and even the eye—could be lost. Most ophthalmologists use antibiotics before, during, and after cataract surgery to minimize this risk. Surface inflammations or infections usually respond well to medication. An infection that may develop within the eye quickly, even a day after surgery, needs immediate attention and treatment.

Intraocular inflammation (swelling within the eye, not due to infection), which occurs in response to the surgery, is usually a minor event that responds to postoperative steroids.

Though uncommon, a slight leak in the incision in the cornea may occur, creating a greater risk for infection inside the eye, as well as other problems. If this occurs, the doctor may apply a contact lens or a pressure bandage over the eye to promote healing but, sometimes, the wound has to be reclosed with additional stitches.

Pronounced *astigmatism*—irregular curvature of the cornea, which will cause blurring of vision—may also develop in some individuals after surgery, due to swelling of the tissue or too-tight stitches that pull on the cornea and distort its shape. After the eye has healed from the operation, the swelling diminishes and any sutures may be cut, which usually corrects the astigmatism. In selected cases, cataract removal can relieve preexisting astigmatism as incisions may be designed to change the cornea's shape.

Bleeding within the eye is another potential problem. It rarely occurs because the smaller incisions enter the eye in the clear cornea, in front of the blood vessels, and no blood vessels are cut inside the eye. However, even bleeding caused by the larger incisions may stop automatically without causing any damage. Hemorrhaging from the *vascular choroid*—the thin membrane in the middle layer of the eye between the sclera and retina—is a rare but serious complication and may be the cause of permanent vision loss.

Another possible complication from cataract surgery is *secondary glaucoma*—a rise in internal eye pressure. It's usually temporary, and may be caused by inflammation, bleeding, adhesions, or other factors that increase the *intraocular* (eyeball) pressure. Glaucoma medications can usually control the pressure, but it sometimes requires laser or other surgery. *Retinal detachment,* a serious condition in which the retina separates from the back wall of the eye, occurs infrequently but requires surgical repair. (*See* page 140.)

On occasion, tissues of the macula may swell one to three months after cataract removal. This condition, called *cystoid macular edema,* is characterized by the blurring of central vision. An ophthalmologist can diagnose it with special testing, and can usually treat it successfully with medication. In rare cases, the implant may become displaced. You might then notice blurred vision, glare, double vision, or fluctuating vision. If it seriously impedes vision, your ophthalmologist can reposition or remove the implant, or replace it with another lens.

In 30 to 50 percent of all cases, the *posterior capsule* (the skin of the old cataract left in the eye to support the implant) becomes cloudy some time after surgery, again causing blurred vision. Referred to as a *secondary* or *after cataract,* this does not mean the cataract has grown back; it's merely a fogging of tissue membrane. If the condition inhibits clear vision, it can be treated with a technique called *YAG* (yttrium-aluminum-garnet) *capsulotomy.* In this procedure, the ophthalmologist uses a laser (*see* "Fixing Eyes with a Flash of Light," page 72) to create an opening in the center of the opaque capsule to allow the passage of light. Quick and painless, requiring no incision, it can be done in an ophthalmologist's office or outpatient clinic.

EYE OPENER

Even if your cataract surgery is considered a success, you still might not see as well as you'd like. Other eye problems, such as glaucoma, macular degeneration, or damage to the retina from conditions like diabetes can still hinder your vision, but cataract surgery might still

*be worthwhile if some degree of your precataract vision
is restored.*

FIXING EYES WITH A FLASH OF LIGHT

In the *Star Wars* movies, Jedi knights deftly wield lasers called *light sabers* to ward off enemies. In the real world, lasers have more constructive uses and, when handled by skilled ophthalmologists, can be used to treat and repair diseased eyes. The word *laser* is actually an acronym for Light Amplification by Stimulated Emission of Radiation. It refers to the narrow, concentrated beam of light created when an electric current is sent through a special substance. The laser's color and name depend on the material used: A blue-green laser comes from the gas argon; a red or yellow light from the gas krypton; and invisible infrared light from YAG (yttrium-aluminum-garnet). Different wavelengths of light are required for treating various eye diseases.

The eye is particularly responsive to laser therapy because of its clear optical tissues. Lasers are used to treat the eyes in two ways. *Thermal lasers* convert light to heat to seal leaking or bleeding blood vessels (as in some types of age-related macular degeneration), to destroy tumors and other abnormal tissue, to secure retinal tears, and to treat some types of glaucoma. *Photodisruptive* (cold) lasers work like a knife, using a light beam to cut or carve out tissue. Where applicable, laser surgery may be the preferred mode of treatment. It's less invasive than traditional surgery, has no risk of eye infection, has fewer complications, and can be performed on an outpatient basis.

LASIK, the newest and most popular form of refractive surgery, is a cross between laser and conventional surgery, and is increasingly being used to correct *myopia* (nearsightedness) to reduce or eliminate the need for eyeglasses. In LASIK, an acronym for *laser in situ keratomileusis,* the doctor uses a blade to cut a flap in the outer layer of the cornea and a laser to reshape the cornea's middle layer. The laser allows the surgeon to accurately remove molecules of the cornea, so that it's reshaped to a flatter curvature, which corrects the refractive error, allowing light to focus directly on the retina. The big advantage of LASIK over other laser surgeries is a shorter recovery period. With LASIK, recovery is generally only a few days at most, as opposed to several days to a few weeks for more conventional laser surgeries. *Photorefractive keratectomy* (PRK), for example, involves removing the surface layer of the cornea by gently scraping and using a computer-controlled laser to reshape the stroma (the thick middle layer of cells in the cornea). LASIK is a more comfortable procedure, and it can also be used to correct hyperopia and astigmatism.

POSTSURGERY: WHEN TO CALL YOUR DOCTOR

Although cataract surgery is generally successful, complications can occur. Contact your doctor immediately if you experience any of the following symptoms after surgery:

- Loss of vision
- Pain that over-the-counter pain medication doesn't relieve
- A significant increase in eye redness
- Light flashes or several new spots (floaters)
- Nausea, vomiting, or excessive coughing

Preventing Cataracts

There is no sure way to avoid developing a cataract. However, because of the link between UV radiation and cataracts, always wear sunglasses and a hat or visor when outdoors. Be especially careful to wear your sunglasses when you're in the mountains, on the beach, and by the swimming pool. In or near the water, everyone gets a double whammy of ultraviolet radiation: the harmful rays from above and those angling from below, reflecting from the water. At higher elevations, the sun's rays are also more dangerous for your eyes, because they're more concentrated. In general, it's a good idea to wear sunglasses and a hat any time you're spending time outside, no matter where you are—even on hazy or overcast days (UV rays can seep through clouds), and on sunny days that aren't so warm. Don't be fooled. You can't see or feel ultraviolet radiation, but it's there, potentially harming your eyes, and it can be powerful. (For more information on choosing the right sunglasses, *see* "Invest in the Right Sunglasses," page 175.)

In addition to protecting your eyes from the sun, there is growing evidence that antioxidant vitamins may play a role in cataract prevention by capturing free radicals, which form unstable molecules that are believed to degrade proteins in the eye's lens. (Exposure to UV radiation and the body's own metabolic processes create free radicals, which damage tissue through oxidation.) In a 1994 study at Harvard University of 17,744 male physicians, those who took multivitamin supplements had a decreased risk of cataract and cataract extraction. Another study found a lower incidence of cataracts among people who took vitamin A and beta-carotene supplements; vitamin E has similarly been associated with reduced risk of cataracts. Though the evidence is not yet strong enough to recommend that everyone take antioxidant supplements, talk to your physician about whether supplement use is appropriate for you. In the meantime, eat plenty of fruits and vegetables, which contain an abundance of antioxidant vitamins. For more information on how your diet may protect you from cataracts and other eye diseases, see chapter 8.

Summary

☛ *Cataract*—the clouding of the eye's lens that results in distorted vision, and even vision loss—is a common condition that typically begins in late middle age, but doesn't usually affect vision until one's mid-sixties.

☞ Cataract surgery, which involves removing the eye's natural lens and replacing it with an artificial one, is one of the most common and successful surgeries performed in America today.

☞ Symptoms of cataract include blurry, cloudy, or dim vision; glare from bright lights; double or multiple vision; distorted images; increasing nearsightedness; declining night vision; and/or frequent changes in your eyeglass or contact lens prescription. If any of these symptoms occur, see an eye doctor promptly for a full examination.

☞ When vision loss associated with cataract affects one's lifestyle, it's time to talk to a doctor about cataract surgery. Cataract surgery is the only effective cure for cataracts. Drugs, eye drops, changing your diet, or new eyeglasses won't reverse the problem.

☞ In recent years, cataract surgery has become more refined. In most cases, it's performed under local anesthesia on an outpatient basis, and lasts less than thirty minutes. Still, it's not without risks.

☞ In addition to age, many factors may contribute to the development of cataracts, including heredity; diet; exposure to the sun's harmful ultraviolet rays; eye injuries; medications, such as corticosteroids; and health problems, such as diabetes.

5

Glaucoma: The Stealth Sight Stealer

Like a thief in the night, glaucoma can snatch sight silently. Nearly four million people in the United States have a chronic form of the disorder, but at least half of those who have glaucoma don't know they have it. Like cataracts, glaucoma is usually painless, and progresses in the initial stages without symptoms. The National Glaucoma Research Foundation estimates that about 50 million people worldwide suffer from impaired vision and/or blindness from the disorder. *Glaucoma* is actually a group of diseases characterized by excessive fluid pressure in the eye, which can damage the *optic nerve*—a bundle of more than one million nerve fibers that connects the *retina,* the light-sensitive layer of tissue at the back of the eye, with the brain. Good vision depends on a healthy optic nerve. In many cases, by the time vision loss from glaucoma is apparent, cells in the optic nerve have already been irreparably damaged and vision is gone forever.

Glaucoma is a major cause of blindness, and threatens two percent of the population over age forty, and becomes even more common with age. However, if glaucoma is caught and treated early through regular routine ophthalmology checkups, vision can almost always be spared.

Types of Glaucoma

Although twenty-five to thirty types of glaucoma exist, those described here are the most common.

Chronic Open-Angle Glaucoma

Chronic open-angle glaucoma, also called *chronic glaucoma,* accounts for more than 90 percent of all glaucoma cases. According to the National Eye Institute, glaucoma affects about 3 million Americans; it's estimated that half of those afflicted with glaucoma don't know they have it, due to the lack of early symptoms. Glaucoma strikes African-Americans most frequently. Most prevalent in people over sixty, glaucoma also tends to run in families.

According to the National Eye Institute, roughly 120,000 Americans are blind from this particular chronic form of the disorder. The name *chronic open-angle glaucoma* comes from the fact that the angle in the *anterior* (front) chamber of the eye remains open. For some reason that researchers don't fully understand, the *aqueous humor*—the fluid in that front chamber—drains too slowly. This leads to fluid backup and a gradual but persistent elevation in eye pressure, which can ultimately damage the optic nerve and cause vision loss if not caught in time and controlled by medication.

More specifically, the aqueous humor circulates through the pupil into the front compartment of the eye, nourishing the lens and lining cells of the cornea, the clear outer covering of the eye. The aqueous humor then drains out of the eye through Schlemm's canal via the *circular trabecular meshwork,* a sievelike drainage system of porous tissue, before being reabsorbed into surrounding blood vessels. As more aqueous humor is produced, excess fluid is eliminated through the trabecular meshwork to keep a healthy balance of pressure in the eye. (*See* Figure 6.) The process works continuously as part of normal vision.

In open-angle glaucoma, the drainage system breaks down, and the outgoing fluid flows too slowly through the meshwork, or not at all. Consequently, the fluid can't leave the eye as it should, and backs up like water in a clogged sink. As a result, the internal pressure in the eye rises. This, in turn, puts stress on the optic nerve, which is responsible for transmitting visual signals to the brain, which then translate into images. If the pressure continues, the nerve fibers that carry the optical messages die, and vision starts to fade. Nerve fibers on the outer edge are affected first, which is why those with glaucoma typically develop blind areas at the edges of their field of vision. If left untreated, your peripheral vision gradually closes in, until the cells supplying central vision are killed off. Loss of vision may also result when the tiny blood vessels that feed the retina and optic nerve cannot deliver the blood into the eye because of the elevated pressure.

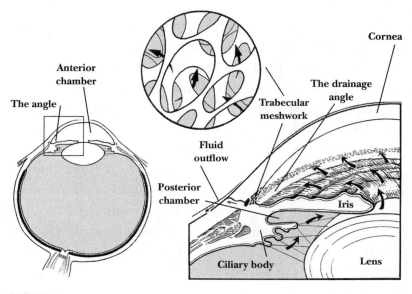

FIGURE 6

Glaucoma: In a healthy person, the ciliary body continuously produces aqueous humor. The fluid bathes and nourishes the interior of the eye, then drains through the trabecular meshwork into small blood vessels. If this sievelike meshwork is blocked, aqueous humor accumulates and pressure increases. Glaucoma occurs when the elevated pressure is high enough to compress and injure small blood vessels and the optic nerve; this can lead to vision loss and blindness if the disease is not treated early.

Acute Closed-Angle Glaucoma

A less-common form of glaucoma, which primarily affects far-sighted individuals in their thirties and over, *closed-angle glaucoma,* also called *acute glaucoma* or acute-angle-closure glaucoma, is caused by a rapid increase in intraocular pressure. In acute closed-angle glaucoma, the pressure in the eye rises rapidly if the angle between the iris and cornea is narrow enough to allow the peripheral iris to block the drainage system, the trabecular meshwork. Anything that causes the pupil to dilate, such as dim lighting, some medications, and even dilating eye drops given before an eye exam, can cause the iris to block fluid drainage in some people. When this form of the disorder occurs, the eyeball quickly hardens, and the sudden pressure causes pain and blurred vision.

EYE OPENER

According to the National Eye Institute, glaucoma accounts for 4.5 million visits to physicians each year.

Low-Tension Glaucoma

Low-tension glaucoma involves optic-nerve damage typical of glaucoma, but at normal eye pressures. The diagnosis is nearly always made after there has been some vision damage, because there are no early symptoms and no way to test for it. After other possible causes of the optic nerve damage and visual loss have been eliminated, lowering the normal pressure even further by medication and/or surgery will usually stabilize the condition.

Congenital Glaucoma

This is a rare condition, present at birth and often inherited. It's attributed to a structural defect in the drainage angle, and is frequently found in both eyes. Congenital glaucoma usually responds to early surgery, and sometimes to medication.

Secondary Glaucoma

Secondary glaucoma may develop as a result of some other eye problem, such as chronic inflammation, eye injury, advanced cataract, certain eye tumors, or as a complication of another medical illness, such as diabetes or lupus, *vascular occlusion* (blockage) in the eye, or even because of the use of systemic medication, such as prednisone or other similar medications.

Symptoms of Glaucoma: Open Angle

Unfortunately, chronic open-angle glaucoma—the kind in which pressure gradually rises in the eye—is insidious and may advance with few or no symptoms. You won't feel the increasing pressure in your eye, and may not notice blind spots and diminishing peripheral vision until late in the disease. Unfortunately, it's at this point that most people seek treatment. Occasionally, sufferers may be alerted that something is awry when they repeatedly need new eyeglass prescriptions, or have trouble adjusting to the dark. However, these symptoms generally occur in advanced stages of the disease; because the chronic form of this irreversible disease may not announce itself until it has done considerable harm, it's crucial to have regular eye exams and routine testing for glaucoma. Left untreated, glaucoma can lead to limited tunnel vision and eventual blindness.

Symptoms of Glaucoma: Closed Angle

Initial symptoms of closed-angle glaucoma, which may only

last a few hours before a full-blown attack occurs, include severe pain, nausea, colored halos around lights, eye redness, and blurry or slightly decreased vision. Then, there may be rapid vision loss and throbbing pain in the eye. This type of glaucoma, which usually affects only one eye, can progress slowly or suddenly without symptoms.

If you see or feel any symptoms of closed-angle glaucoma, contact your eye doctor immediately. Closed-angle glaucoma is a medical emergency, because optic nerve damage and irreparable vision loss can happen within hours.

In general, to protect yourself from glaucoma, make an effort to have your eyes examined every two to four years by an optometrist or ophthalmologist if you're between age forty and sixty-four, and every one to two years by an ophthalmologist after age sixty-five. Be especially diligent if you have any of the risk factors mentioned for glaucoma, such as diabetes, a family history of glaucoma, or if you've had an eye injury earlier in life. Don't wait until your vision blurs or you experience other symptoms.

If you're diagnosed with glaucoma, you will need to see the eye docotor as often as four times a year to monitor the effectiveness of treatment, and to be sure the glaucoma is stable. Visual loss and blindness from glaucoma can be prevented if the disease is discovered before the optic nerve is severely damaged.

What Causes Glaucoma?

Although increased pressure within the eye, which ultimately damages the optic nerve, is the primary cause of glaucoma, that's not always the case. Some people who have normal intraocular pressure develop optic-nerve damage and vision loss, a condition referred to as normal or low-tension glaucoma. Similarly, some people with elevated intraocular pressure, a condition often called ocular hypertension, never develop glaucoma and visual loss. (These rare cases are best monitored closely by an ophthalmologist.) Clearly, there are other factors at play besides ocular pressure that cause glaucoma; research is underway to discover underlying causes of the disease.

In any event, if you have glaucoma and don't receive prompt and effective treatment, your vision will gradually deteriorate from the edges inward, until you can no longer see in your central line of sight and blindness develops. The damage that occurs in glaucoma is irreversible.

Who Gets Glaucoma?

No one is immune to glaucoma, but some people are more likely to develop the disease than others. The Baltimore Eye Survey, supported by the National Eye Institute, found that, by age seventy, about one in fifty Caucasions has glaucoma. In African-Americans, the problem is more severe, as by age seventy, one in eight has the disease. In general, you're at increased risk for glaucoma if you:

- are older than age forty
- are of African-American descent
- have a family history of the disease
- have elevated *intraocular* pressure (internal eye pressure)

☛ have had a past serious eye injury

Diabetes, severe nearsightedness, or farsightedness, routine use of steroid drugs, a history of anemia and shock, and/or a Scandinavian, Irish, or Russian background, are also associated with increased risk of one or more types of glaucoma. Just why glaucoma seems to appear as people get older isn't clear but, like other bodily processes that wind down with age, the eye's drainage system also seems to become less efficient at doing its job.

GLAUCOMA AND OBSTRUCTIVE SLEEP APNEA

It's estimated that about half of all normal-tension glaucoma patients and one-third of all primary open-angle glaucoma patients suffer from *obstructive sleep apnea* (OSA), a disorder in which sleep is interrupted because air can't flow into or out of your nose or mouth, although you continue to make efforts to breathe. Besides glaucoma, OSA is associated with irregular heart beat, high blood pressure, heart attack, and stroke. Snorers are often suspected OSA sufferers, as are those who are overweight. Although research on the connection between OSA and glaucoma is not conclusive, if you have been diagnosed with OSA, it's especially important to see your ophthalmologist regularly to be tested for glaucoma.

GLAUCOMA: WHAT TO WATCH FOR

With open-angle glaucoma, you may not experience any symptoms, which is why it's important to see your eye doctor regularly for routine eye exams. If you notice any of the symptoms listed below, see your eye doctor immediately:

- difficulty focusing on close work
- loss of peripheral (side) vision
- not being able to adjust to a darkened room
- multicolored rings or halos around lights
- the need to change eyewear prescriptions frequently

In the closed-angle form of glaucoma, symptoms are much more defined. They include:

- blurred vision
- considerable eye pain
- rainbow haloes around lights
- sensitivity to light
- headaches
- nausea (only when associated with the visual symptoms)
- vomiting (only when associated with the visual symptoms)

EYE OPENER

Closed-angle glaucoma is a serious condition and can cause blindness in a relatively short time, sometimes

within hours. Don't wait to seek treatment. If you experi-
ence any symptoms, see your ophthalmologist immediately.

Diagnosing Glaucoma

To test for glaucoma, the ophthalmologist evaluates fluid pressure in the eye through tonometry by measuring the force necessary to indent the eye. With the air-puff technique, a stream of air is blown gently against the eye. A more accurate measuring device, called an *applanation tonometer,* is placed on or near the eye, which has been anesthetized, to gauge the eye's resistance. (For more information on detecting glaucoma, *see* "Measuring Eye Pressure," page 46.) Normal pressure is considered to be in the range of 12 to 21 millimeters of mercury (mm Hg) but, as mentioned earlier, people whose *intraocular* (internal eye) pressure falls in this range may still develop the disease. Likewise, those who have slightly elevated pressure may not be destined to get glaucoma: How much stress the optic nerve can withstand differs for each person and each eye. To confirm the presence of the elevated pressure, the doctor may repeat the tonometry test, as the fluid pressure in the eye may vary at different times of day.

A thorough evaluation of the optic nerve is necessary, and should be done as part of a routine eye exam. It's best done with a dilated pupil, which allows the doctor to better see the back of your eye to examine the optic nerve. The doctor uses both a slit lamp and an ophthalmoscope to look for any deterioration of the optic nerve. If the optic disk, the front surface of the optic nerve, is affected by glaucoma, a condition known as *cupping* may be observed. That is, the optic disk may appear indented, and its color—normally pinkish yellow—may turn pale and more yellow, because the advancing disease has hindered blood flow to the area.

Gonioscopy

If your doctor suspects glaucoma, he may perform an examination called *gonioscopy,* which examines the eye's *drainage angle*—the area between the iris and the cornea—for blockage. This procedure involves placing a special contact lens on the surface of an anesthetized eye. The lens has special mirrors and facets that, when studied through a slit lamp, give a detailed view of the corner of the eye and show whether the drainage angle is open, narrowed, or closed.

Fundus Photography

Fundus photography, which may be used to produce three-dimensional pictures of the *optic disk*—the front surface of the optic nerve—will provide a baseline for later comparisons of the disk. A change in the appearance of the optic disk in patients with glaucoma usually means that pressure hasn't been controlled, and an increase in therapy is needed. An ophthalmologist also may use *laser polarimetry,* a technique that uses a beam of laser light to measure and follow the thickness of the retinal nerve fiber layer just before they come together to form the optic nerve that carries the light to the brain.

Once you've been diagnosed with glaucoma, your eye doctor may also perform more general tests to determine the extent of your vision loss, if any. Each year, glaucoma patients typically undergo two to four examinations that involve measuring visual acuity, the optic disk, and the pressure in the eye. The doctor will also check peripheral vision to find out if there is lost side vision, and may perform other tests done at selected intervals to establish the stability of the disease or to note deterioration.

Medications for Glaucoma

Most types of glaucoma, including chronic open-angle glaucoma, can't be cured. Unfortunately, vision lost to the damage of glaucoma can't be regained. (It is best to detect and treat the glaucoma before any visual loss has occurred.) However, glaucoma can be controlled to keep the disease from doing further damage. The goal of therapy—a lifetime commitment for both the patient and the physician—is to control eye pressure and stop the disease from progressing.

Open-angle glaucoma treatment usually begins with topical medications—eye drops or sometimes ointments—that patients apply one to several times a day to help fluid better drain through the trabecular meshwork or to decrease the eye's production of aqueous humor. Depending on the severity of the glaucoma, multiple drops and, sometimes, pills may be required. Unfortunately, glaucoma medications can be expensive and may cause side effects, such as headaches, lower pulse and blood pressure, fatigue, respiratory problems, allergic reactions, impotence, and even a change in eye color. Most ophthalmologists begin with the lowest effective dose to minimize potential side effects and the cost of the drops. If side effects occur, consult with your eye doctor for advice on alternative treatment.

Types of Medications
The following classes of drugs are listed in the order in which an ophthalmologist is most likely to prescribe them to treat glaucoma. However, the doctor will personalize treatment based on the individual characteristics of each patient. Depending on the severity of glaucoma and your medical history, for example, your physician may prescribe these drugs in a different order, or may use two or more of the drugs in combination. (See the Appendix for specific drugs.) The more commonly used medications tend to have fewer and less severe side effects than those less commonly prescribed.

Prostaglandins: This topical drug is commonly used because it requires only one application per day. It lowers internal eye pressure by removing aqueous humor through the *uveal tissues,* which includes the iris, ciliary body, and the *choroid,* the inner lining of the eye. Prostaglandins may cause allergic reactions, *uveitis* (inflammation) within the eye, blurred vision due to *macular edema* (swelling of the macula, the central area of the retina), headache, and fatigue. In addition, for some people, this medication has startling cosmetic effects that include causing lashes to grow longer and thicker and changing the iris color from blue or hazel to brown. An ophthalmologist may thus be less likely to prescribe this drug for someone with hazel or blue eyes.

Beta blockers: These topical eye drops, similar to beta blockers used to treat some types of heart disease, are commonly prescribed for glaucoma, and are used once or twice daily. Topical beta blockers lower pressure in the eye by reducing the amount of aqueous humor produced by the eye's *ciliary body*, which is just behind the iris. This class of medication is usually well tolerated with continued use, but has potentially serious side effects. In a small percentage of patients, when the drug enters their system, they may experience a slowing of the heart rate, a sense of mental and physical lethargy, a decrease in libido (in men; the effect on women's libido has not been researched), and/or a worsening of asthma. Patients with chronic lung disease may experience serious breathing problems. Topical beta blockers may be used by patients who are also taking the drug systemically (not topically) for heart disease, but it's important to notify both your ophthalmologist and physician that you're doing so. Topical side effects include allergy and eye irritation.

Alpha-2 agonists: This medication, used two to three times a day, lowers *intraocular* (internal eye) pressure by both decreasing production of aqueous humor and increasing the fluid outflow from the eye. It may cause allergic reactions, eye irritation, dry mouth, general fatigue, and other symptoms.

Carbonic anhydrase inhibitors (CAIs): This class of medication, which can be administered either orally or topically, decreases eye pressure by reducing the amount of aqueous humor produced in the eye, as do beta blockers. CAIs may cause prominent side effects, including numbness and tingling in the hands and feet, excessive urination, loss of appetite, drowsiness, lethargy, depression, anemia, and allergic reactions. The eyedrop form of CAIs may have fewer side effects than the pills, but even the drops can cause an allergic reaction, a bad taste in the mouth, and the other side effects that the pills cause. If you have been prescribed CAIs, it's a good idea to be aware of these potential side effects and to keep your eye doctor updated.

Miotics: *Miotics,* the oldest of the currently used medications for glaucoma, improve the drainage system capacity when applied as eye drops. Pilocarpine, carbachol, and echothiophate iodide, a stronger miotic, may produce blurred vision by decreasing the size of the pupil. This may be especially troublesome if you have cataracts. These medications may produce nearsightedness in young glaucoma patients, limit night vision, and cause chronic inflammation in the eye or even retinal detachment. One of the miotics may also cause cataracts. Side effects may also include diarrhea, sweating, and other symptoms. Miotics are used infrequently, because their side effects on vision are more common and troublesome than those of many of the other glaucoma medications.

Adrenergics: These drops contain either epinephrine or dipivefrin, which becomes *epinephrine* (otherwise known as *adrenaline*) when absorbed into the eye. Adrenergics decrease the secretion of aqueous humor and increase the eye's outflow via the *trabeculum,* the eye's meshlike drainage system. Epinephrine, which is naturally secreted by the adrenal glands, is the agent that causes the heart to beat fast and palpitations to occur when you're frightened or angry. When used in the eye to increase the eye's outflow of fluid, it may cause similar systemic effects, such as heart palpitations. Topical local symptoms within the eye include the dilation of the pupil, allergies, and redness (a common cosmetic side effect).

Hyperosmotic medication: In the case of acute glaucoma, *hyperosmotic medication* (which reduces pressure in the eye by pulling fluid from the eye into the internal eye blood vessels, then out of the eye with the normal blood flow of the general vascular system), may be taken orally or injected.

EYE OPENER

There's a growing list of alternative treatments for glaucoma, including herbs, such as bilberry extract, meditation, and biofeedback to lower intraocular pressure and improve blood flow to the eye. While these natural therapies are often based on sensible ideas about good health, there have been few controlled studies to support or discredit their effectiveness. In general, avoid using them in lieu of conventional treatment that has been proven based on numerous clinical studies. If you'd like to try a natural therapy, tell your eye doctor. Despite their questionable status, some doctors recommend them in conjunction with proven therapies.

Side Effects of Glaucoma Drugs

Although the symptoms and side effects from glaucoma medications appear formidable, in actual practice, most don't occur in the average patient. Most people tolerate these medications either alone or in combination to treat glaucoma. If you have problems with any medication, tell your eye doctor. You may be able to switch to a different dosage, or even to a new drug. Also, remember that glaucoma medications are potent drugs. If you're taking other medications for other conditions, even something as simple as a decongestant, be sure to tell your ophthalmologist and pharmacist, to avoid adverse drug interactions.

EYE OPENER

Some beta blockers used to treat glaucoma may lower levels of HDL ("good") cholesterol and increase the risk of heart disease, the nation's number-one killer. If you're taking beta blockers for glaucoma, be sure to tell your personal physician, particularly if you have heart disease or are at increased risk for the condition due to elevated cholesterol, your age, or other factors, such as a family history of heart disease.

Minimizing Side Effects

Although topical eyedrops help to control pressure in the eye, they may have accompanying side effects, such as dizziness or breathing trouble, which could limit or prohibit their continued use. These side effects may affect the eye itself, causing stinging, burning, or redness, or they may be systemic, as the drops enter the bloodstream after they're absorbed through the nose and throat. You can avoid absorbing too much of the medication into your system by turning your head outward when you apply your eyedrops. This tactic lets the excess liquid run to the outer reservoir of your eye instead of allowing it to pool in the inner corner, where it can be absorbed into the nose and throat. Another trick: After you apply your eyedrops, compress the tear duct leading into the nose, by placing your index finger deep within the inner corner of your eye; this allows more of the medicine to stay in your eye and prevents it from entering your nose and throat.

EYE OPENER

If eyedrops prove difficult for you, talk to your eye doctor about alternatives. You might be able to use gels or ointments. Another treatment option is to insert a medicated disk with a time-release mechanism in the lower conjunctiva sac (the clear membrane that covers the front portion of the white of your eye) between the lid and the eyeball. However, these drug delivery systems tend to be more expensive than traditional medications, and are often more cumbersome.

Applying Eyedrops

Not to be confused with over-the-counter eyedrops for common eye irritations, eyedrops for glaucoma are serious medicine. Here's a step-by-step guide to applying topical eyedrops, so you can routinely get the proper amount of medication into your eye.

1. Before applying your eyedrops, wash your hands.

2. To apply the medicine, bend your neck back so that you're looking up at the ceiling; turn your head slightly outward, and use one finger to pull down your lower eyelid to create a small pouch for the medicine.

3. Without letting the tip of the bottle touch your eye or eyelid, squeeze just one drop of the medicine into the space between your eye and your lower eyelid. If you squeeze more than one drop, you're probably wasting medicine, wasting money, and possibly getting too much medicine into your system.

4. After the drop has entered your eye, close your eye, then press a finger deep within the inner corner of your eye and hold for several minutes. Gently closing your eye will ensure the medicine spreads over its surface.

5. After you've put eyedrops in your eyes, wash your hands. While capping the medicine, try not to let the tip of the bottle touch anything, such as a table or countertop, to avoid contamination.

6. If you need to take more than one eye medicine, wait ten to fifteen minutes before applying any subsequent medicine, to allow each medicine to be absorbed into your eye. Different drops placed in the same eye too soon will each dilute the concentration of each medicine. Generally, the drops should be used every twelve hours if prescribed twice a day, every eight hours if prescribed three times a day, and so forth.

Sticking with Your Medication Routine

Because glaucoma has no symptoms, you may be tempted to stop taking your medication or forget to take it. However, to prevent glaucoma from doing further damage, it's important to use your eyedrops and/or take pills for glaucoma, as long as they help to control your eye pressure for as long as your doctor recommends. Even if the disease is stable and symptoms disappear, don't stop taking your medicine unless your doctor advises it.

Regular exams are equally important because, without an exam, it's not possible to tell whether fluid pressure in your eye is in a safe range, or if your visual field is slowly changing. Patients with chronic glaucoma are commonly examined two to four times a year to ensure that medication is effectively controlling eye pressure, and that their vision is being preserved. Work with your physicians and other caregivers to ensure that you can properly maintain your glaucoma therapy. If you have questions about your drugs, trouble following your treatment plans or difficulty applying the drops, mention them to your doctor, and ask for advice and solutions.

Glaucoma Surgery: When Drugs Don't Help

If the pressure in your eye can't be controlled with the maximum tolerated medication, your ophthalmologist may advise that you undergo laser or conventional glaucoma surgery. The ophthalmologist, who commonly deals with these issues, will doubtless have literature or web sites for you to consult, and will be prepared to discuss the reasons for performing the operation, as well as the risks and benefits of surgery. (For more information, you may wish to do your own research. "Resources," starting on page 229, is an excellent reference tool.) The following types of surgery for glaucoma are currently available.

Laser trabeculoplasty: When medications aren't totally effective, your doctor may recommend *laser trabeculoplasty,* a form of laser surgery that helps fluid drain out of the eye in open-angle glaucoma. (See Figure 7.) Laser surgery can't reverse the damage that's been done, but it can prevent glaucoma from progressing, in many cases. The ophthalmologist usually performs the procedure in her clinic or office, using a high-energy laser beam to burn tiny spots onto the surface of the eye's *trabecular meshwork,* which is part of the eye's anterior chamber drainage system. The doctor makes about fifty burns in half of the trabecular circumference; the burns stretch the existing holes in the meshwork to allow fluid to flow out of the eye more freely.

Before the procedure, which is typically painless, the doctor numbs the eye with drops, which allow a special contact lens with mirrors to be placed on the eye. As you sit in a comfortable position at the slit lamp, the ophthalmologist applies the contact lens as your other eye fixes on a target. You may see flashes of green or red light as the laser is focused and fired. The treatment takes less than one-half hour. The doctor will check the internal eye pressure after treatment before allowing you to go home. The doctor will also prescribe drops for minor inflammation, along with the regular glaucoma medicines, and will schedule several followup visits to monitor your eye's intraocular pressure.

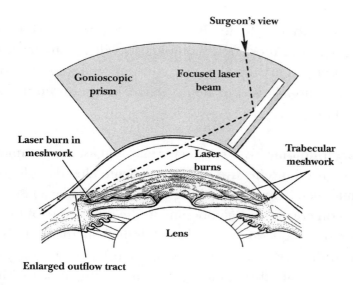

FIGURE 7

Laser trabeculoplasty for glaucoma: If glaucoma cannot be controlled with drugs that reduce the intraocular pressure, a doctor may recommend *laser trabeculoplasty*. In this procedure, the surgeon uses a high-energy beam of light to produce small burns on the trabecular meshwork while viewing the eye through a prism. The procedure improves the outflow of aqueous humor from the eye. A silt-lamp microscope and a contact lens allow the ophthalmologist to get a detailed view of the angle where the iris, cornea, and sclera meet, and to focus the laser on the tissue.

You may experience blurred vision and sensitivity to light for a day or two after the operation, but you shouldn't feel any pain or discomfort.

While laser surgery is often helpful, the benefits may not be permanent: If it's only partially successful, your doctor may need to perform the procedure again on the other half of the trabecular circumference. Moreoever, some patients don't respond to laser surgery. After about two years, more than half of all patients experience a rise in eye pressure to unsafe levels and will require conventional surgery. Still, most ophthalmologists will recommend trying laser surgery first, because conventional surgery carries the additional risks of hemorrhage, infection, and other problems.

Laser iridotomy: Your eye doctor may suggest this technique, which is often effective in treating acute closed-angle glaucoma, even before prescribing medication. Using a laser, the surgeon creates a small opening in the outer edge of the iris to help the aqueous humor better drain from the back chamber to the front chamber. (*See* Figure 8.) The ophthalmologist can create this opening without making an actual incision in the eye, an advance over the older, prelaser procedure, which required surgical incision and scissor excision of the iris. Laser iridotomy cures closed-angle glaucoma in many patients, making drug treatment unnecessary. Topical medication and/or conventional surgery may be warranted, however, if the eye has suffered permanent damage before the iridotomy is performed, such as the iris permanently adhering to the trabecular meshwork, blocking the flow of aqueous humor out of the eye.

Conventional incisional surgery: Conventional surgery is used by ophthalmologists when medications or laser surgery aren't successful in treating chronic open-angle glaucoma, or when acute closed-angle glaucoma has gone untreated and caused permanent damage. Conventional incisional surgery, also known as *filtering surgery* or *trabeculectomy,* creates a new drainage system when the trabecular meshwork is either scarred or no longer functions. It can be done as outpatient surgery.

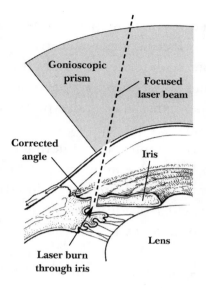

FIGURE 8

Laser iridotomy for glaucoma: The early stages of closed-angle glaucoma may be relieved by a laser iridotomy. The surgeon uses a laser to make a small opening in the edge of the iris to increase drainage of the aqueous humor from the posterior to the anterior chamber.

In the most common procedure, the *trabeculectomy,* an eye surgeon opens a flap of tissue to form a new passageway, so that fluid can drain from the front chamber of the eye to a space created beneath the conjunctival tissue under the upper lid. This filtering bleb helps bring pressure in the eye down, and eye fluid is reabsorbed into the bloodstream.

In an alternative technique, used in scarred tissue, the surgeon implants a special plastic valve to provide drainage for outflowing eye fluid. Filtering surgery is successful in 80 to 90 percent of patients; the other 10 to 20 percent can usually undergo further surgery, which usually improves eye pressure adequately. Most patients can eliminate or reduce their use of glaucoma medication after filtering surgery. This type of surgery is an involved procedure, so ask your ophthalmologist to refer you to an eye surgeon who has the proper experience and expertise if your ophthalmologist doesn't do this type of surgery. The surgery isn't without risks or complications; filtering blebs may leak fluid and may be susceptible to infection. The surgery may also lead to blurred or decreased vision from retinal swelling at the macular of the retina, and can also cause the development of cataract.

Cyclodestructive surgery: In this procedure, the surgeon uses a cool laser or a thermal (heat) laser to treat glaucoma by destroying the cells in the eye's ciliary body (the vascular structure behind the iris whose surface cells produce aqueous humor). The surgeon applies a probe, usually on the surface of the eye, and treats the secreting cells of the ciliary body through the intact *sclera* (the white of the eye). This reduces the amount of aqueous humor formed in the eye. Cyclodestructive surgery is useful when other methods of glaucoma control haven't been successful.

EYE OPENER

If you're diagnosed with advanced glaucoma, your eye doctor will likely recommend a course of therapy to preserve and prolong your vision based on your unique patient characteristics, which may include your race. According to the National Eye Institute of the National Institutes of

Health, African-American and white patients with advanced glaucoma may respond differently to surgical treatments for the disease. Research suggests that African-American patients with advanced glaucoma not responding well to medications benefit more from a surgical treatment regimen that begins with laser surgery, while Caucasians benefit more from one that begins with trabeculectomy (conventional incisional surgery). However, filtering surgery is usually successful for all patients.

Preventing Glaucoma

Because early diagnosis and treatment remains the key to preserving sight, the surest way to prevent glaucoma-related blindness is to know the risks, and to have your eyes examined regularly. If you have risk factors for glaucoma, such as being over the age of sixty, having a history of glaucoma in your family, or a having had a past eye injury, your eye doctor is likely to monitor three things: *intraocular* (internal eye) pressure, your optic nerve, and the quality of your peripheral vision. If you've been diagnosed with glaucoma, your vision may be protected for a lifetime if your glaucoma is properly treated.

EYE OPENER

As you read this, research studies are underway to better diagnose, monitor, and treat glaucoma. In the past, such studies have led to new ways to diagnose and monitor glaucoma, as well as a variety of new drugs to reduce intraocular pressure, which, in turn, reduces pressure on the optic nerve. However, even those medications don't necessarily stop the disease from progressing. Many people still continue to have vision loss due to glaucoma, because there are mechanisms other than elevated intraocular pressure that lead to loss of vision.

A likely suspect is the untimely death of cells in the optic nerve. On the horizon may be a new type of drug for glaucoma that prevents the early death of nerve cells. This medication, which is already being used in Europe and the United States to treat patients with Parkinson's disease, diabetic neuropathy, and AIDS-related dementia—all of which involve nerve cells that die in an untimely way—may help keep optic nerve cells alive, thereby preserving vision. If you've been diagnosed with glaucoma, stay tuned. Government organizations, such as the National Eye Institute of the National Institutes of Health, and others, are working hard to develop new drugs and therapies that may treat glaucoma and thereby protect and improve visual health.

Summary

☞ Glaucoma is a major cause of blindness, and threatens 2 percent of the population over age forty, becoming even more common with aging. If glaucoma is caught in its early stages through routine vision checkups, vision can almost always be saved.

☞ Typically, those with glaucoma develop blind spots at the edges of their vision, which can gradually close in, eventually leading to blindness.

☞ Risk for glaucoma is increased for those who are older than age forty, have a family history of the disease, have elevated intraocular pressure, are of African-American descent, or have had a serious eye injury in the past. Those at risk should see an eye doctor yearly.

☞ *Open-angle glaucoma,* among the most common forms of the disease, gradually increases pressure within the eye, perhaps because the natural drainage system in the eye is clogged. The increased pressure stresses the optic nerve; if nerve fibers in the optic nerve die, vision will fade.

☞ A less common form of glaucoma, *closed-angle glaucoma,* is marked by a sudden increase in internal eye pressure, because fluid in the front chamber of the eye can't drain. Closed-angle glaucoma is a medical emergency because optic-nerve damage and irreparable vision loss can occur within hours.

☞ An eye doctor should be seen promptly if it becomes difficult to focus on close work; side vision disappears; and/or eyes lose their ability to adjust to a darkened room. All are potential signs of open-angle glaucoma. Other warning signs include blurry vision, considerable eye pain, rainbow haloes around lights, headaches, nausea, or vomiting. All may be signs of closed-angle glaucoma, a medical emergency.

☛ Being diagnosed with glaucoma doesn't mean future blindness. Medication and surgery is available to help prevent the disease from progressing to complete vision loss.

☛ Unfortunately, there's no way to prevent glaucoma other than knowing the risks and regular eye examinations.

6

Protecting Your Sight from Age-Related Macular Degeneration

Unlike glaucoma, which in its earliest stages, affects peripheral vision, age-related macular degeneration (AMD) strikes at the heart of the eye's vision center—the macula, which is the area on the retina responsible for sharp central vision. (*See* Figure 9.) Those with AMD experience blurred vision and the inability to see things in front of them clearly. In some cases, vision loss is rapid and dramatic.

If you're affected by AMD, you may develop a blind spot in the middle of your field of vision that may increase in size as the disease progresses. This blind spot can impact the ability to perform day-to-day activities that require straight-ahead, or central, vision, such as reading, sewing, driving, and recognizing faces. (Peripheral vision doesn't change.)

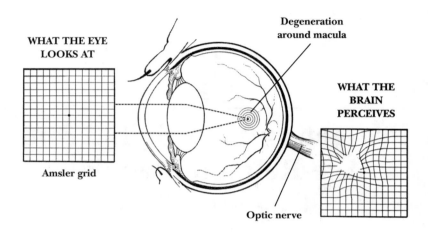

FIGURE 9

Age-related macular degeneration: The leading cause of legal blindness in people over fifty-five, it results from the deterioration of the light-sensitive cells of the *macula,* the central part of the retina. People may first experience blurred or distorted vision and see straight lines as wavy. As the condition progresses, they will notice a black or dark space at the center of their visual field. In demonstrating the defect to the patient, an ophthalmologist may use an Amsler grid test. The patient focuses on a dot on a grid. If the lines near the dot appear wavy, macular degeneration may be responsible. Direct examination of the retina and fluorescein angiography will confirm the diagnosis.

A potentially devastating disorder, AMD is the most common cause of legal blindness in people over age fifty-five. The prevalence of AMD increases with age. More than 13 million Americans have the disease, and 5 percent of people age sixty-five and older experience some visual impairment because of it. Yet, for some sufferers, there's still only limited treatment. Despite extensive research, as well as the introduction of photodynamic therapy for one type of the disease, there is no laser, medical, or surgical treatment that works for the most common form of the disease.

EYE OPENER

Because AMD spares peripheral vision, AMD patients rarely go totally blind.

Types of AMD

The disease occurs in two main forms: *dry* and *wet.* The vast majority of afflicted (90 percent) have the dry or *atrophic* type, in which small yellowish deposits called *drusen* form and start to break down the *photoreceptors* (light-sensing cells) in the macula area of the retina. Dry AMD may affect only one eye at first, presenting itself with gradual distortion of the visual field and blurring of the vision in the central line of sight. It's common for the second eye eventually to fall victim as well (the same holds true for cataract and glaucoma). One of the first signs of dry AMD may be distorted vision while reading. As cataracts also may reduce vision when reading, you should seek early evaluation to be sure what is causing the problem. Remember, some types of AMD can be helped by laser—but only *early* in the course of the disease.

Wet AMD, which is more severe and less forgiving, results when abnormal blood vessels develop and extend under and into the retina, toward the macula, like tree roots growing under a sidewalk. These new vessels are fragile and prone to leak fluid and blood, which injure tissue and photoreceptor cells, rapidly damaging the macula and distorting vision, and possibly causing severe vision loss in a short time. Wet AMD progresses more rapidly than dry AMD, and almost always occurs in those who already have dry AMD. According to the Food and Drug Administration, if wet AMD isn't treated promptly, the majority of those with the disease will become functionally blind within two years. Although wet AMD accounts for only 10 percent of all AMD cases, it accounts for 90 percent of all cases of legal blindness in macular degeneration patients. Both forms of the disease may cause a blind spot in the central field of vision.

EYE OPENER

Younger people may develop different kinds of macular degeneration, some inherited and some acquired.

Causes and Risk Factors

Scientists still don't know why AMD develops, nor do they know exactly why the macula deteriorates. Various theories are being explored. Aging itself is a major risk factor: People in their fifties have only a 2 percent chance of developing AMD; that risk jumps to 30 percent in those older than seventy-five. Women (who tend to outlive men) get the disorder more often, as do people with a family history of the disease. Race is also a factor; Caucasians are more likely to lose vision from AMD than African-Americans.

Other factors that increase your risk include smoking, exposure to bright sunlight and UV radiation, having light-colored eyes, being farsighted, and/or having hypertension, high cholesterol, or coronary artery disease. Some researchers also believe that deficiencies in certain vitamins and minerals may leave you more vulnerable to AMD. For example, studies suggest that not getting enough of the following nutrients increases the risk of AMD: the antioxidant vitamins C and E; the mineral zinc, which exists in trace amounts in the body but is concentrated in the eye; and carotenoids lutein and zeaxanthin, which are stored in the dominant pigments in the macula. For more information on diet's relationship to eye disease prevention, *see* "More Reasons to Eat Your Five a Day," page 163. Meanwhile, ongoing research continues to focus on causes—such as hereditary factors, diet, and environmental conditions—with the ultimate hope of preventing AMD.

What to Watch for: Dry AMD
Although symptoms vary, those with the dry form of AMD often first experience:

- blurred vision
- difficulty with reading or distinguishing faces

Be aware of these symptoms and report them to your doctor. Dry AMD doesn't cause any pain. Nonetheless, as the condition advances, you may notice a blind spot at the center of your visual field. With time, this area may enlarge and hinder sight. However, if you have AMD in only one eye, you may not realize that you have any vision loss, because there's a tendency to compensate with your healthy eye.

EYE OPENER

While central vision can be severely affected, AMD doesn't affect the peripheral retina. Those with AMD don't go totally blind from even the most severe forms of the disease. Still, AMD can severely limit your vision and keep you from living a full and active life.

What to Watch For: Wet AMD

Be alert for any of the following symptoms. If you experience one or more, report them to your doctor immediately:

☞ Distorted vision, in which straight lines appear wavy and shapes looked deformed, or the center of your vision appears more distorted than the rest of the scene. These are among the earliest signs of wet AMD caused by leaking blood vessels, which raise the position of the macula to distort it.

☞ Blurred vision.

☞ Faded colors.

☞ Difficulty reading (this AMD symptom may go away when you brighten your reading light).

☞ Difficulty distinguishing faces.

☞ A small but growing blind spot or whiteout area in the center of your field of vision.

Like dry AMD, wet AMD is painless. Patients do not experience symptoms, such as redness, irritation, itching, or tearing from AMD.

Diagnosing AMD

You may have signs of AMD before your sight is affected, but only an eye examination will detect them before you experience permanent vision loss. A routine eye exam that involves dilating your pupils with eye drops to allow your eye doctor to get a better view of the back of your eye should uncover AMD. The exam should also include an acuity test, to measure how well you see at different distances and under different light with the best corrective glasses; in some cases, the vision specialist may also administer a color test to see how well the retinal cone cells in your eye are operating.

A complete eye exam will rule out or identify coexisting eye diseases, such as cataract or glaucoma. Your doctor may suspect dry AMD if there are clusters of *drusen,* small yellow deposits that build up under the macula or clumps of pigment, which are visible through an ophthalmoscope. These lesions on the macula are an early sign of AMD. However, there are other diseases that can also cause drusenlike spots.

The Amsler Grid Test

The Amsler grid test, using a pattern that looks like a checkerboard or graph paper, is another crucial part of the eye exam, because it can identify the distorted vision associated with AMD. This is especially important if you have wet AMD, which may be treatable in the early phases of the disease. (If damage is in the center of the macula, however, it may be untreatable.)

The test is simple: Simply look at the central spot on the Amsler grid. If the lines near the dot appear wavy, AMD may be to blame. If your doctor suspects wet AMD, you'll likely undergo *fluorescein angiography*. In this test, a special dye is injected into your arm; eventually, it travels to the blood vessels in your retina. Images are taken to reveal the passage of the fluid through your retinal blood vessels. The procedure helps your ophthalmologist determine if leaking vessels in your eye can benefit from laser treatment. If the damage or leakage is too extensive, your doctor may rule out laser surgery and recommend optical (low-vision) aids instead. Once permanent damage has occurred, low-vision aids may help you function better, but changing the glasses will not fully compensate for the loss of vision.

Treating Dry and Wet AMD

There are several treatments available that may help slow or halt the progress of AMD. Unfortunately, no treatment currently exists for dry AMD. However, a trial study, sponsored by the National Institutes of Health, will evaluate *pro-*

phylactic (preventive) laser to patients with dry AMD who appear to be at greatest risk of getting worse. Unfortunately, results are still several years away.

Because dry AMD progresses very slowly, you may be able to manage your daily routines quite well, even with some central vision loss. If the condition worsens, special low-vision aids, such as magnifying lenses, or closed circuit televisions that "read" regular print, then enlarge it on a monitor can help you maintain your quality of life. *See* "Living with Low Vision," page 147.)

EYE OPENER

Among the more promising treatments for dry AMD on the horizon is a threshold, or low-intensity, laser therapy, in which patients undergo a mild laser procedure that removes drusen (bothersome yellow deposits).

Wet AMD

Laser surgery, called *laser photocoagulation,* is effective for some people with wet AMD. In this procedure, the doctor aims a *thermal* (heat) laser beam at leaky blood vessels to cauterize or seal them to prevent further fluid seepage. Patients reap the most benefits when the procedure is done on newly formed vessels that haven't yet encroached on the fovea, the central part of the macula. However, this technique isn't a cure, and usually doesn't restore vision that has already been destroyed; if successful, it merely halts the disease from progressing.

As with other laser surgeries, laser photocoagulation—sometimes performed in multiple treatments—takes about thirty minutes, and can be done in a doctor's office. (The surgery is often helpful but, in about half the cases, the condition recurs, and more laser treatments may be needed.) After laser photocoagulation, you may experience some mild discomfort and sensitivity to light. Frequent checkups will be scheduled, at which time your doctor may repeat the fluorescein angiography to assess the status of the blood vessels. Like many medical procedures, laser photocoagulation isn't risk free. It's possible to experience permanent vision loss in the form of blind spots following treatment. Speak to your eye doctor about your individual risks.

Visudyne Therapy

Among the newest treatments for wet AMD is *Visudyne therapy,* which is part of an emerging new platform of technology called *photodynamic* therapy, which uses light-activated drugs to treat a wide range of medical conditions—from cancer and heart disease to autoimmune conditions and eye diseases, including in wet AMD. Visudyne therapy was approved by the Food and Drug Administration in 2000. It may be especially appropriate for wet AMD patients who aren't eligible for laser photocoagulation.

Visudyne therapy is a two-step, twenty-minute process that can be done in a doctor's office. During the procedure, Visudyne is injected into a vein in the arm over a ten-minute period. During the next five minutes, the drug travels through the body, then accumulates in the abnormal blood vessels in the eye. Subsequently, the eye doctor will activate the drug by shining a cool laser into the eye for roughly ninety seconds. Visudyne therapy affects the retina, without damaging surrounding healthy eye tissue, by producing a highly energized form of oxygen that causes abnormally growing cells to die. Visudyne therapy may stop vision loss but rarely restores vision; more often, it simply slows retinal damage and any decline in vision experienced due to wet AMD. To preserve your vision, usually more than one Visudyne treatment per year is needed.

If you undergo Visudyne therapy, stay out of the sun for two days after treatment; you'll want to avoid exposing your skin or eyes to direct sunlight or bright outdoor light. Your eyes may be extrasensitive to light. Speak to your eye doctor for more information about Visudyne therapy, and the dos and don'ts associated with the procedure.

EYE OPENER

Transplanting healthy cells into the retina to replace diseased cells is another approach being explored for both wet and dry AMD; the results on animals are promising, but the treatment is experimental and rarely performed on people. Research on gene therapy is also underway, with the hope of some day substituting normal retinal genes for damaged ones. Additional surgeries include removing new blood vessels from beneath the macula in wet AMD, and relocating the macula to other areas of more healthy underlying tissues.

BEWARE OF SHAM TREATMENTS

There are countless so-called treatments for AMD, many in the form of nutritional supplements, advertised in magazines and on the Internet and other media that promise to restore vision, or cure or prevent the condition. They may even be allegedly recommended by eye doctors. Buyer beware. No matter how frustrated you are with AMD, keep in mind that these kinds of treatments haven't been adequately tested for safety or efficacy by the Food and Drug Administration. In addition, they may be expensive and usually aren't covered by health insurance. If you're considering trying a treatment you've read or heard about, first consult your eye doctor.

Detecting AMD

Although AMD can't be cured, detecting AMD in its early, most treatable, stages is important to prevent the retina from further deterioration. It's critical that those between forty and sixty-four have their eyes examined by an optometrist or an ophthalmologist every two to four years, and that those over age sixty-five have their eyes examined every one to two years by an ophthalmologist.

Home Monitoring

If you're diagnosed with dry AMD, you can monitor your condition and whether it's progressing to wet AMD by testing yourself at home with an *Amsler grid*, which has a pattern resembling graph paper with a dot in the middle. Keep the paper on the refrigerator door or other convenient location. Routinely test each eye. Wet AMD may be present if the lines near the spot look wavy. If you've already had laser surgery, regular checks of the Amsler grid may alert you to the recurrence of leakage in blood vessels.

To use the Amsler grid, hold it twelve to fifteen inches away from your eyes, in good light. With your reading glasses on, cover one eye. Look at the center dot and note whether all lines of the grid are straight or if any areas are wavy, blurred, or dark. Repeat with the other eye. If any areas are wavy, blurred, or dark, contact your ophthalmologist.

EYE OPENER

If you have already lost some of your vision to AMD, low-vision aids can help maximize whatever sight is left. Ophthalmologists can prescribe appropriate aids and provide referrals to agencies that offer support and assistance to the visually impaired. (See "Living with Low Vision," page 147.)

Preventing AMD

While there is no surefire way to prevent age-related macular degeneration, you can take steps that may delay the onset of the disease, or reduce its severity. Because smoking can accelerate AMD damage, quitting smoking is an important preventive step. (For tips on stopping smoking, *see* "There Has Never Been a Better Time to Stop Smoking," page 171.) Wearing a hat, and sunglasses that block the sun's blue ultraviolet wavelengths—thought to promote AMD—may also help protect you. (For more information, *see* "Invest in the Right Sunglasses," page 175.)

There's also some evidence that certain nutrients may help prevent macular degeneration. Middle-aged and older people may benefit from diets rich in fresh fruits and dark leafy greens like spinach or collard greens. Supplements of antioxidant vitamins C and E may also help. (Be careful when taking supplements—too high a dose of some vitamins can be harmful. Talk with your doctor before starting an over-the-counter vitamin supplement.) There is also some research indicating that a diet high in saturated fat may increase your risk of developing AMD. Though the verdict is still out, reducing saturated fat in your diet is healthful in several ways, and might help prevent AMD. The most benefit is likely gained from eating a well-balanced diet with fruits and leafy greens. Although a number of studies have looked at supplements, no clear benefit has been definitively shown for AMD. For more information on diet's relationship to eye-disease prevention, *see* chapter 8.

Summary

☛ Age-related macular degeneration (AMD) is a common, painless age-related eye disease in which the *macula*, the tiny area of the eye's retina that's responsible for sharp central vision, deteriorates. Those with macular degeneration can't clearly see things in front of them, and may find it difficult to focus on close work, read, sew, or drive.

☛ The risk of AMD increases with age, family medical history, race, and lifestyle factors. To help prevent the onset of the disease or reduce its severity, don't smoke; wear sunglasses, and, on sunny days, a wide-brimmed hat; fine-tune dietary intake to ensure it contains plenty of fruits and vegetables. The antioxidants they contain may help preserve vision.

☛ The Amsler grid test, a pattern test that looks like a checkerboard, is an important part of identifying and monitoring AMD. To detect wet AMD, simply look at the central spot on the grid. If the lines near the dot appear wavy, AMD should be suspected.

☛ Laser surgery is available to treat some forms of wet AMD; no treatment exists for dry AMD.

7

Other Common Eye
Disorders of Later Life

Although the passage of time leaves people more vulnerable to cataract, glaucoma, and age-related macular degeneration, you may be lucky never to experience serious eye disease. As you age, however, you may encounter some changes in your vision, or other vision problems less critical than these disorders.

Presbyopia: Ready for Reading Glasses

Presbyopia, the slow loss of the ability to see close objects or fine print, is one of the first signs that your eyes are showing their age. Suddenly, you may need to hold menus and newspapers at arm's length to read them. *Presbyopia,* the Greek word for "old sight," is a loss in the eye's focusing ability that may start as early as the late thirties, but typically begins between age forty and forty-five, gradually worsening over the next three decades.

Presbyopia is not a disease, and it can't be prevented. Although it seems to strike overnight, the actual loss of lens flexibility takes place over many years. More of a nuisance than anything else, presbyopia occurs when the aging lens thickens and becomes more rigid and, therefore, less efficient at bending, or accommodating changes in near and distant focus. An accompanying lag in the function of the *ciliary eye muscle*, a circular muscle that surrounds the lens, contributes to the difficulty in seeing small print. Normally, the ciliary muscle expands and contracts, changing the curvature of the lens to accommodate for near or distant vision. However, with presbyopia, the lens stiffens and becomes less able to change its shape. As a result, close vision becomes blurry, because images focus behind, instead of on, the retina.

Blurred near vision that leaves your eyes tired and strained provides an early hint of presbyopia's arrival. After reading or doing other detail work, it may be difficult to see distant objects clearly. You may get headaches. The problem may be more pronounced in the evening when you're tired or when you're reading in low light. The condition occurs regardless of whether you're nearsighted, farsighted, or astigmatic. With astigmatism, your vision may be blurred at any distance.

EYE OPENER

Presbyopia happens to everyone sooner or later. According to the National Eye Institute, presbyopia is the most common disorder of the aging eye.

Although everyone is a presbyopia patient waiting to happen, presbyopia may hit farsighted people sooner than those who are nearsighted. If you're nearsighted, you may be able to overcome presbyopia when it first develops by simply taking off your glasses to read. Eventually, however, as your presbyopia worsens and the lens of your eye becomes stiffer, you may need corrective lenses just like everyone else with the condition.

When it comes time for corrective lenses, your choices in eyewear are among the types that follow.

☞ **Reading glasses:** If you've had good vision before your presbyopia developed, you'll probably only need reading glasses to magnify printed material and correct the problem. Many drugstores and supermarkets carry magnifying reading glasses that may help in the early stages. Don't go to the reading glass counter blindly. First, see your ophthalmologist and get your eyes examined. To help you choose the right reading glasses for your needs, your eye doctor can recommend how much power you need for magnification. Overall, you may be better off with prescription reading glasses that offer a closeup correction; they may be more comfortable and offer you a sharper image than do over-the-counter glasses.

If you're already wearing glasses or contact lenses because you're farsighted, nearsighted, or have astigmatism, you'll need a new prescription that corrects your presbyopia in addition to the other refractive errors you have. Your eye doctor will likely prescribe bifocals, trifocals, progressive lenses, or contact lenses.

EYE OPENER

The effects of presbyopia usually stabilize by about age sixty, when the eye's focusing ability has virtually disappeared as the ciliary muscle does no work and your near vision is totally dependent on glasses. Until then, you may need to change your eyewear prescription frequently to keep seeing clearly and comfortably. To monitor your presbyopia, be sure to visit your eye doctor for an eye exam every two to four years if you're forty to sixty-four and every one to two years if you're age 65 or older.

☞ **Bifocals:** If you already wear corrective lenses, you may need bifocals or two pairs of glasses—one for distance and one for close work. Bifocals contain two lenses—an upper lens that corrects the distance vision and a lower lens that corrects the close vision. With bifocals, you can avoid taking off and putting on your glasses for various tasks, since you now have two prescriptions on one lens. Bifocals come in two styles, those with a visual horizontal line and those that are ground so that the line doesn't show (progressive). Progressive, lineless bifocals change gradually from distant correction at eye level to reading correction at the bottom level. If you've never worn bifocals before, you might start out with the progressive ones. But if you're already wearing lined bifocals, you may want to stick with them. Some people prefer the sharp contrast you get with regular lined bifocals.

If you see distorted or wavy images or can't find a distance where images are clear, you may have the wrong prescription, or your glasses may not be fitted properly. As with any type of glasses, bifocals that slide down your nose or lenses that aren't centered correctly within the frame won't allow you to see clearly.

☛ **Trifocals:** By the time you reach age fifty or so, you may lose most of your ability to naturally focus on objects that are in the mid-distance range, such as your computer screen or the name tag of someone at a party. That's when trifocals come into play. (Those with presbyopia who wear bifocals often graduate to trifocals.) Trifocals contain three lenses—an upper lens to correct nearsightedness, a lower lens to correct farsightedness, and a small midsection of lens located just above the bifocal segment on the eyeglass lens to make corrections for middle-distance vision. In essence, trifocals combine correction for close, middle, and distance vision all in one.

☛ **Progressive lenses:** These provide a seamless focus by blending the distance, intermediate, and near focusing power. When fitted well there is *no* distance from infinity to near vision that is *not* in focus. Even trifocals have areas of blurring. The vision is good in the upper portion to right and left. The only blurring is to the right and left of glasses for near—only straight ahead is clear—but one doesn't read through the sides of one's bifocals or progressives.

☛ **Monovision contact lenses:** These are another option for correcting presbyopia, especially for those who wish to avoid eyeglasses. With monovision contacts, you wear a contact lens to correct near vision in one eye and, if necessary, a lens for correcting distance vision in your other eye. The eye that's set for close vision will be slightly blurred for distance. Although it sounds complicated, most people do adjust to monovision contact lenses, and don't even notice that each eye is responsible for a different aspect of their vision. Patients may have glasses to use over the contact lenses to allow both eyes to be clear at distance or near vision.

☞ **Bifocal contact lenses:** If you're bothered by a distant or near blur that may occur with monovision, bifocal contact lenses are an option to investigate. They work in much the same way as bifocal eyeglasses: They have two corrective powers on one lens, one for distance and one for near vision. Like bifocal eyeglasses, you can get them in lined form, in which there's an obvious separation between the two prescriptions. You can also get them as progressive lenses that have the prescription seamlessly blended on the lens. Bifocal contacts are available in daily-wear soft and rigid gas permeable materials and in disposable, extended-wear, and planned-replacement form. Bifocal contacts aren't for everyone. The contact may move or spin when you blink, which can affect your quality of vision. It takes time for most wearers to adjust to bifocal contact lenses.

☞ **Modified monovision:** With this option, you wear a bifocal contact lens in one eye and a contact prescribed for distance in your other eye. The theory is that you have both eyes clear for distance and have one eye for reading.

☞ **The monocle contact lens:** Another lens option for presbyopia correction is to wear a single contact lens, which is focused for reading and other close work, in one eye only.

Obviously, there are plenty of choices when it comes to correcting presbyopia, with more options available all the time. For more information on corrective eyewear and what's right for you, speak to your eye doctor.

LASIK Surgery for Presbyopia

Laser-Assisted In Situ Keratomileusis (LASIK) surgery is another option that has been approved by the Food and Drug Administration that may help reduce your dependency on contacts or glasses. With this refractive laser surgery, presby-optic patients undergo a monovision procedure in which one eye is operated on to correct distance vision, and the other eye is operated on to correct near vision. The goal is to have the patient experience both good uncorrected distance as well as near vision when the two eyes work together. LASIK surgery, also called "flap-and-zap" surgery isn't a cureall. Afterward, you may still need reading glasses for very small print or when doing close work for long periods.

LASIK surgery permanently changes the shape of the cornea, the clear covering of the front of your eye, using an *excimer laser,* an ultraviolet laser that removes tissue from the cornea. During LASIK surgery, a knife, called a *microker-atome,* is used to cut a flap in the cornea. A hinge of tissue is left at one end of the flap. After the flap is folded back to reveal the stroma, the middle section of the cornea, pulses from a computer-controlled laser vaporize a portion of it and the flap is replaced.

Although the success rate is very high (95 percent satisfaction with LASIK), LASIK surgery has its risks. Results may not be lasting, and temporary or permanent vision loss is possible. You may need more than one surgery to get the desired results. When considering this surgery, be sure to do your homework, taking into account the potential risks, limitations, and alternatives available, depending on your situation. For more information, speak to your ophthalmologist. You may also wish to consult the FDA's Web site, www.fda.gov, which discusses the pros and cons of the procedure. If your eye doctor doesn't perform LASIK, ask for a referral to an experienced eye doctor who does. Avoid going to an eye center that promotes LASIK surgery by promising 20/20 vision or your money back. With LASIK surgery, there are never any guarantees.

Eyelid Problems

Age can affect the muscles and skin of the upper and lower eyelids in several ways. Often the problem is simply cosmetic but, in other cases, it may interfere with your vision or irritate your eyes.

Ptosis: Drooping Eyelids

Like other parts of your body that respond to gravity over time, such as your skin, one or both of your eyelids may start to sag as their muscles lose their strength. An eye injury, neuralgic problems, or disease, such as diabetes or the neuromuscular disorder *myasthenia gravis,* can also precipitate the condition. *Ptosis* (pronounced "toe-sis") occurs when the upper eyelids droop more than normal. The condition may affect one or both eyes and may impair your vision.

Although drooping of the upper lid is more of a cosmetic concern than a medical one, it can become troublesome if the lid is so lax that it covers, or partially covers, the pupil. If you think you suffer from ptosis, see your ophthalmologist. A medical exam is necessary to discern the underlying cause. Ptosis resulting from a disease, such as myasthenia gravis or eye inflammation, will usually respond to treatment for that particular condition. However, if a droopy eyelid is merely unattractive, or if it interferes with your vision and isn't caused by a treatable disease, surgery may help.

To correct ptosis, your eye doctor may advise you to undergo a procedure called *blepharoplasty* (ptosis surgery)— reconstructive eyelid surgery that removes excess tissue, lifts the lid, and restores vision. This surgery, which usually leaves nearly invisible scars, tightens muscles and lifts the loose skin into a normal position. It's usually performed under a local anesthetic on an outpatient basis.

Before undergoing *blepharoplasty,* be sure to have your eye doctor fully document your condition. A complete eye evaluation may be necessary, including *visual field charting* (mapping your central and peripheral vision), to qualify the surgery as medically necessary and therefore eligible to be covered by health insurance. Many insurance plans will pay for ptosis or blepharoplasty surgery only if it functionally limits your vision.

Your ophthalmologist can easily diagnose whether you have a functional problem as well as a cosmetic one.

EYE OPENER

If you wish to avoid ptosis surgery, you do have another option: eyelid crutches, which attach to eyeglasses to hold up the drooping eyelid. They are rarely used, however.

Blepharochalasis

In a different but related condition, blepharochalasis, the skin of the lid begins to droop, not the muscles of the entire lid, as in ptosis. When this happens, the skin loses elasticity and may sag, creating new skin folds that can actually droop over the lashes and, as in ptosis, block the upper field of vision by covering the pupil. Blepharochalasis may be surgically corrected through blepharoplasty, whether it's a cosmetic or a functional problem. But, as with ptosis, many insurance plans will pay for blepharoplasty surgery only if your condition limits your vision.

Blepharoplasty is usually done on an outpatient basis under local anesthesia, and typically takes one to three hours; most surgeons use local anesthesia, leaving the patient awake. Some surgeons, however, prefer to use general anesthesia, in which case, the patient is asleep throughout the operation. If you think you suffer from blepharochalasis, see your ophthalmologist.

BLEPHAROPLASTY (EYELID SURGERY)

When you undergo the procedure, the surgeon will typically make incisions that follow the natural lines of your eyelids. Through these incisions, the surgeon will remove excess fat and trim sagging skin and muscle before closing the incisions with fine sutures.

After surgery, your eyes may feel tight and sore as the anesthesia wears off. You'll likely be asked to keep your head elevated for a few days, and to use cold compresses to reduce swelling and bruising. The stitches will probably be removed a few days after surgery. For the first few weeks, you may experience excessive tearing, light sensitivity, and blurred vision. Be sure to wear sunglasses when you go outdoors. Within two to three days, you should be able to watch television or read. Within a week to ten days, you'll probably be ready to go back to work and resume your normal activities, although you may be advised to avoid strenuous activity for three weeks or so. For six months or more after surgery, your scars may remain slightly pink. In time, however, rest assured that they'll fade to a faint, often undetectable, line.

Ectropion: Drooping Lower Lids

Ectropion—the sagging and the outward turning of the lower eyelid and eyelashes—causes aging eyelid muscles to relax to the point at which the lower lid no longer comes in contact with the eyeball. As a result, the eyelids can't meet properly and the margin of the lid may thicken. The eye may also tear excessively, since the lower lid isn't there to help tears spread over the eyeball during blinking and the lower tear duct opening pulls away from the eye. Ectropion may also cause eyes to become red and irritated, since the cornea and *conjunctiva*—the thin membrane that covers the eye—are constantly exposed. The disorder may involve one or both eyes.

If you think you suffer from ectropion, see your ophthalmologist. Often, in mild cases, no treatment is needed. You may simply be advised to use artificial tears or wear a special plastic eye shield designed to keep moisture in the eye at night. However, if the symptoms or appearance of ectropion are especially bothersome, surgery designed to tighten the lower eyelid and the surrounding muscles can usually correct it. The goal of the procedure is to secure the lower lid so that it rests more closely against the eyeball. After the surgery, you may need to wear an eye patch overnight, and apply an antibiotic ointment for a few days.

Entropion: Inward-turning Lower Lids

This condition, which is the opposite of ectropion, causes the upper or lower eyelid to roll inward toward the eye, due to aging eye tissues. As a result, the skin of the eyelid and the eyelashes rub against the cornea and conjunctiva, irritating the eye. Because eyelashes and the skin of the eyelid constantly rub against the cornea, entropion can lead to scarring and ulcers of the cornea, blurry vision, excessive tearing, crusting of the eyelid, mucous discharge, and the feeling that something's constantly in the eye.

If you think you suffer from entropion, see your ophthalmologist. Like ptosis and ectropion, this disorder can be corrected with a relatively simple outpatient surgical procedure. In most cases, your doctor will tighten the eyelid and surrounding tissue. Sometimes, in mild cases, your doctor may simply advise you to tape the lower lid to your cheek nightly so the lid margin and lashes are in the proper position. If your doctor recommends this technique, he will instruct you as to how to do it properly.

Dry Eye Syndrome

Aside from helping us express emotions, tears coat the eye with layers of water, *lipids* (oil), and mucus. They wash away foreign matter, protect against infection, and keep the eye comfortably lubricated. As you age, tear production naturally declines and what sometimes results is *dry eye syndrome*—irritated moisture-challenged eyes that frequently burn or feel painfully scratchy. Dry eye syndrome leaves the cornea feeling like a sandy beach; eyes may sting and burn. Sometimes, it may be mild and not require treatment. Some people with dry eye syndrome become sensitive to light, have trouble wearing contact lenses, find it difficult to cry when they're upset, and/or have blurred vision that can affect their daily lives.

Paradoxically, with dry eye syndrome the eye sometimes tears in response to irritation caused by lack of normal lubricating tears. However, these dry tears are of poor lubricating quality. Adding proper lubrication with artificial tears may actually decrease total tear production but, in this case, quality is more important than quantity. (*See* Appendix: "Drugs Used to Treat Dry Eye Syndrome," page 215.)

Dry eye syndrome affects most people over age sixty-five. It's estimated that roughly 10 million Americans suffer from the condition. Dry eye syndrome is more common in women and may start in middle age, at menopause. Studies suggest that dry eye syndrome may be associated with the cycle of reproductive hormones. People with allergies are more susceptible to this malady; it is also associated with systemic diseases, such as lupus or rheumatoid arthritis. A shortage of tears is also one of the symptoms of Sjögren's syndrome, a disorder of the immune system that results in chronic dryness of the mouth, eyes, and mucous membranes. For more information on these and other eye-related conditions, *see* "Protect Yourself from Diseases Associated with Vision Problems," page 198.

Dry Eye Syndrome: What to Watch For

- a persistent gritty sensation in your eyes
- becoming intolerant of contact lenses
- not being able to cry when you're upset
- a burning sensation in your eyes when the humidity is low or air pollution is high

Treating Dry Eye Syndrome

If you suspect you may be suffering from dry eye syndrome, see your ophthalmologist. Your eye doctor can diagnose dry eye syndrome with a slit lamp, and can test the amount of your eye's tear production, if necessary. Treatment frequently involves applying topical drops and ointments that soothe the eye and act as artificial tears. Both the drops and ointments are available without a prescription; they resemble your own tears and contain substances that hold water in your eye. However, some over-the-counter eyedrops for red and sore eyes can actually dry your eyes out further because they contain *vasoconstrictors*, chemicals that constrict the blood vessels in your eye. Choose a brand of artificial tear eyedrops that your ophthalmologist recommends and use it as needed. Although dry eye may be sporadic, chronic sufferers may need to use artificial tear eye drops on a daily basis.

To help keep tears from evaporating, avoid dust, pollen, cigarette smoke, and other pollutants, and stay out of the wind and away from air blasts from hair dryers and air conditioners. On windy days, wear wraparound glasses; when you're swimming, don goggles.

Humidifiers can add moisture to indoor air; to ameliorate dry eye, it's best to keep the humidity in your home between 30 and 50 percent during the winter, and when the furnace is in use. See your ophthalmologist if these measures don't relieve your dry eyes.

In rare cases, when dry eye symptoms don't respond to lubricating eye drops, dry eye can become serious. In these cases, an ophthalmologist can perform a minor surgical technique to insert plugs into the tear drainage ducts of your eyes. Each eyelid has an opening, called a *punctum* on the inside surface of the lid, that allows tears to drain into the nasal passage. Your eye doctor can insert a tiny plug in one or both of these openings to decrease the amount of tears that escape. The plugs prevent natural tears from draining through the opening on the inner corner of your eyelid. As a result, your tears stay on the eye longer.

This simple procedure is painless, and usually takes only a few minutes in your doctor's office. If you have problems with punctal plugs, your eye doctor can remove them in minutes. Alternatively, your ophthalmologist may prescribe special soft contact lenses that hold in moisture, or recommend that you switch to eyeglasses if you wear contact lenses. You may also be advised to wear goggles at night to help your eyes retain moisture, especially if your eyes don't fully close during sleep.

EYE OPENER

If you suffer from dry eye syndrome, you might want to try limiting your caffeine consumption. Caffeine can dehydrate the tissues in your body, including your eyes. Obvious sources of caffeine include coffee (103 mg caffeine per six ounce serving), tea (36 mg per six ounce serving) and cola beverages such as Classic or Diet Coke (46.5 mg per twelve ounce serving), and Mountain Dew (54 mg per twelve ounce serving). Hidden caffeine sources include Dannon coffee-flavored yogurt (44.5 mg per eight ounce serving), green tea (40 mg per six ounce serving), and chocolate (6 mg per one ounce serving).

Floaters

Once you reach your sixties, it's common to often notice occasional gray or black spots, opaque flecks, or cobwebs drifting across your line of vision, particularly when you're looking at a computer or a solid, light background, or reading. These *floaters* are tiny clusters of cells or gel that have separated from the vitreous humor, the clear, jellylike fluid that fills the space inside of your eyes. Floaters typically result when the vitreous humor deteriorates, due to aging. What you're actually seeing is the shadow these little clumps cast on the retina.

About 25 percent of people have vitreous detachments and floaters by their sixties, and 65 percent by their eighties. Floaters also appear more often in those who are nearsighted or have had cataract surgery. In most cases, although annoying, they're harmless. See your ophthalmologist for an examination for an accurate diagnosis, when you first notice floaters. Certain eye diseases or injuries can also cause them. For example, the onset of new floaters that occur suddenly or seem to worsen over time can signal that you may be suffering from a weak, torn retina, detached retina, or other serious eye condition.

Using special equipment, your eye doctor will examine the vitreous humor and retina after giving you special drops to enlarge your pupils. Floaters, accompanied by light flashes with or without blurry vision, also demand a full retinal examination. Floaters can also be small drops of blood from a torn retinal vessel. (*See* "Retinal Detachment," page 140.)

EYE OPENER

If floaters impair your central line of vision, moving your eye by looking up and down may provide temporary relief. Unfortunately these central floaters often come back to the center line of sight but may, in time, disappear. Eye movement causes the fluid inside your eye to shift and propels the floater out of the way, so it disappears spontaneously.

Once your floaters have been checked, you'll have to live with them if they're declared harmless. In most cases, they're likely to diminish gradually over weeks or months, but may not go away completely. In time, you may simply learn to ignore them. Although they can be surgically removed, the risk from surgery is greater than that of the floater itself.

Flashes

Seeing stars or flashes of light—a condition called *photopsia*—is also a common age-related problem. Solitary flashes appear as sparks or minuscule strands of light, almost like streaks of lightning across the sky. They are seen when vitreous gel movement creates traction or tugs on the retina, a common result of aging. When the gel liquifies flashes may repeatedly last for a second or two, being more obvious when you move your eyes or when you're in a dark room. These flashes of light are different from the flashing or zigzag lights of a migraine headache, which some people experience simultaneously in both eyes, sometimes for as long as fifteen to twenty minutes. Generally harmless, flashes require no treatment.

Still, it's wise to consult your ophthalmologist when you first notice flashes, as they could signal more severe retinal complications. It's especially important to visit an ophthalmologist if they appear suddenly—even without floaters—or with any loss of peripheral vision.

Retinal Detachment

So far in this chapter, we've covered the less serious conditions associated with aging eyes. However, this one is different. In some cases, floaters and flashes are signs of retinal detachment. This serious condition results when the retina—the thin sheet of light sensitive nerve tissue lining the inside of the eye, which generates electrical impulses that are sent via the optic nerve to the brain—separates from the back wall of the eye, like wallpaper peeling off a damp wall.

Although anyone can experience retinal detachment, even newborns, you're at increased risk for the disorder if you're over age fifty, if you've had a cataract removed or had significant eye injuries or eye inflammation, if you have a family history of retinal detachment, or if you're nearsighted. (Nearsightedness increases the chances of retinal detachment because the nearsighted eyeball, which is naturally elongated, has already stretched and stressed the retina.) Every year, approximately 20,000 Americans suffer from retinal detachment.

The retina can detach when the vitreous gel pulls on the retina with enough force to tear it, creating a hole. When the retina tears, fluid from the vitreous may pass through the tear and push the retina from the *choroid*, the blood vessel layer of tissue that nourishes the retina. Retinal detachment often causes vision loss, because the detached areas no longer receive the proper nutrition necessary for the eye to see. Once retinal tissue becomes disorganized or scarred with the detachment, the body can't replace it. However, if the rupture is caught and treated early, it may be possible to prevent complete retinal detachment from occurring. Even if the retina fully detaches, it can be fixed, but with less assurance than if it is discovered before complete detachment occurs. That's why it's important to see your ophthalmologist if you experience flashes or the sudden onset of a new floater. When not treated promptly, the retina may continue to detach until it's nearly totally separated from the back of the eye, maintaining only a slim connection at the optic nerve and the ciliary body in the front of the eye. (*See* Figure 10.)

Because the underlying disorder may occur in both eyes, you will need to have each eye thoroughly examined. The second eye may also have retinal degeneration or retinal holes that require treatment.

WHAT TO WATCH FOR: RETINAL DETACHMENT

This serious condition can lead to a permanent loss of vision. Early warning symptoms of retinal detachment may include:

- flashing lights and blurred central vision.
- new floaters that travel across your field of vision.
- Gradual shading of vision from one side, much like a curtain coming down or a shade being drawn in front of your eye. The dark area may occur in any part of your field of vision. If the dark area reaches the center of your field of vision, you won't be able to see fine detail.
- Quick deterioration of sharp central vision; this occurs when the macula detaches.

If you experience any of these symptoms, see your ophthalmologist immediately. Retinal detachment is a medical emergency, and requires prompt urgent treatment. Taking quick action is the best way to increase the chances of restoring your sight. During your eye exam, your eye doctor will dilate your pupils and inspect your eyes with special equipment to determine the extent of the detachment, the location of holes in your retina, and the best way to treat the problem. Several types of surgery are available to treat retinal detachment, depending on the severity of the condition. The goal is to repair any tears or holes in the retina and prevent them from recurring.

Treating Retinal Detachment

Some retinal tears don't require treatment, but most cases of retinal detachment call for surgery to reposition the separated retina against the back wall of the eye. With current methods and prompt treatment, the majority of retinal detachments can be repaired. You may not, however, retain perfect vision, since detachment can damage the retina. If

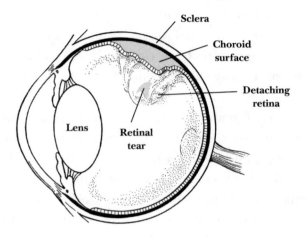

FIGURE 10

Retinal detachment: Degeneration of the retina or pulling on it by the vitreous humor may cause a retinal tear. When this happens, blood may ooze into the vitreous gel, and black spots or floaters will be seen. In some cases, fluid may collect behind the retina, detaching it from underlying tissue and causing a blank space to develop in the person's field of vision. If caught in time, a detached retina can be surgically repaired with no visual loss.

your macula, the central, most sensitive, part of the retina, wasn't affected by the detachment, you're more likely to regain your reading vision. If your macula was harmed, your reading vision may not return. Here are some current treatments for retinal tears and retinal detachment that your eye doctor may recommend.

☞ **Cryopexy:** In retinal tears with minimal or no detachment, your ophthalmologist may repair holes by applying *cryopexy* (freezing probes), that form scar tissue and permanently seal the break, thereby securing the retina to the underlying layer. The procedure is performed on an outpatient basis, using a local anesthetic.

☛ **Laser photocoagulation:** In this procedure, performed on an outpatient basis with a local anesthetic, pinpoints of thermal laser light create tiny burns around any small holes in the retina to weld the retina to the back wall of the eye.

☛ **Scleral Buckling:** If the retina has already started to pull away from the *choroid* (the thin membrane in the middle of your eye), and the gap has filled with fluid, the situation may call for *scleral buckling*, among the most common operations for retinal detachment today. This procedure involves draining abnormal fluid in the eye to allow the retina to fall back against the choroid before sealing the hole. During this intricate procedure, the *sclera* (the white of the eye) is tucked or indented slightly to make better contact with the retina and secured with a silicone buckle sutured around the circumference of the eyeball.

☛ **Pneumatic Retinopexy:** One of the newest methods for repairing retinal detachment, *pneumatic retinopexy* involves injecting a bubble of special gas into your eye. The gas pushes against the area of the retinal tear to block fluid from passing and promote adhesion. If you undergo this treatment, you must avoid flying or traveling to high altitudes until your doctor says the bubble is gone. A rapid rise in altitude can lead to an increase in the size of the bubble and a dangerous rise in eye pressure.

EYE OPENER

If you undergo surgery for retinal detachment, you will

perhaps experience mild discomfort afterward, and need to wear an eye patch for a short time. Once you remove the patch, you may notice that the flashing lights and floaters continue for a while; total recovery may take up to several weeks.

☛ **Vitrectomy:** Some complicated cases, such as detachments with unusually large tears, scar tissue on the retina, excessive blood in the vitreous, or detachments that fail to reattach by other methods, may require that the vitreous humor be removed, a process called *vitrectomy*. In this delicate procedure, the surgeon uses microsurgery to remove the vitreous gel from the eye, which might be causing traction or tugging on the retina. Because the body doesn't regenerate vitreous, a saline solution or other substance similar to the liquid being removed from the eye is inserted as a permanent substitute. A vitrectomy is performed under local or general anesthesia, and can be done on an outpatient basis. In cases where there is a retinal detachment, one of the procedures discussed here is combined with the vitrectomy.

If treated early, 80 percent of vitrectomy patients regain their sight with the first treatment. In other cases, more treatments may be necessary to repair the damage.

Summary

☛ *Presbyopia*—a loss in the eye's focusing ability that may start as early as one's late thirties, occurs when the eye's aging lens becomes more rigid and, therefore, less efficient in bending and accommodating changes for near vision. It's a sign that it's time for reading glasses to magnify printed material and otherwise see close work.

☛ Eyelids can also show signs of age by drooping and possibly impairing vision. In many cases, eyelid surgery can correct the problem.

☛ Dry eye syndrome, the condition in which tear glands don't make enough tears, or make dry tears that don't lubricate sufficiently, is common among those over age sixty-five. Fortunately, lubricating eyedrops often correct the problem, although they may need to be applied several times a day for the rest of the patient's life.

☛ Gray or black spots or cobwebs floating across your line of vision may be nothing more than *floaters*—harmless clusters of cells that have separated from your eye's vitreous humor. They may also be signs of retinal detachment, a potentially blinding condition, in which the retina separates from the back wall of the eye.

☛ If you are very nearsighted, have had an eye injury, or have had cataract surgery, you are at increased risk for retinal detachment, a possibly blinding condition. It's important to see an eye doctor immediately if there is blurred central vision, flashing lights or new floaters traveling across the field of vision, or a gradual shading of vision, like a curtain being drawn in front of the eye. In many cases, retinal detachment can be treated with surgery if it's caught before too much damage has occurred.

8

Living with Low Vision

Usually, impaired vision due to diseases like AMD, cataract, glaucoma, or diabetic retinopathy can't be corrected to normal or even near normal with glasses, contact lenses, medication, or surgery. This noncorrectable vision distortion is referred to by the catch-all terms *low vision,* or *partial vision.* According to the National Eye Institute, there are approximately 14 million Americans—one out of every twenty people—with low vision and 135 million afflicted people worldwide.

Although those with low vision often still have useful eyesight, the condition is often frustrating, because they might not be able to see well enough to perform everyday activities, such as reading the mail, checking pricetags, cooking, watching television, recognizing faces, and crossing the street without help from others. The symptoms may range from blurry vision to more disturbing problems like a complete absence of central vision. There are practical ways to deal with low vision, ranging from learning new ways to perform daily activities to using special equipment, such as the good, old-fashioned magnifying glass or sophisticated computer equipment.

EYE OPENER

Low vision is like a lot of medical conditions: While doctors don't have a cure for low vision, there are plenty of ways to cope and make the most of the remaining eyesight you have.

LOW VISION: WHAT TO WATCH FOR

Many of those experiencing mild reduction of vision aren't aware they have it. According to the National Eye Institute, you may be suffering from low vision if you have trouble doing the following tasks, even with your best correcting eyeglasses:

- recognizing the faces of family members and friends
- doing things that require you to see well up close, such as reading, cooking, sewing, or fixing things around the house
- matching your clothes
- doing activities around the house or at work because the lights seem too dim, no matter how bright you make them
- reading street or bus signs or the names of stores

If any of these sound familiar, see your eye doctor as soon as possible.

In general, the earlier you seek treatment, the more likely it is that you'll be able to preserve the vision you have and continue to lead an active, independent life.

Low-Vision Aids

If you have low vision due to intractable eye disease, in many cases low-vision aids—many of which are simple and inexpensive—can improve your quality of life. Before buying a low-vision aid, such as those described here, it's a good idea to undergo a thorough eye exam with an eye doctor who specializes in low vision, to determine the extent of your vision loss and the type of devices you might need to meet your needs. Once you've been prescribed low-vision aids, you should continue to have regular eye exams to monitor changes in your vision, and to identify the need for new or different equipment. You might also experiment with several low-vision aids for a few months before deciding which ones work best for you.

Low-vision aids generally fall into two categories: optical and nonoptical. Optical aids generally use a magnifying lens to make objects and words appear closer; nonoptical aids are designed to be easier to see or to make use of your other senses, such as your hearing, to perform certain activities. Depending on the low-vision aids you choose, you may need training to help you use them.

Optical Low-Vision Aids

Magnifying lenses: The magnifying lens remains among the oldest and most common way of adjusting to low vision; it magnifies reading material much more than even the strongest prescription eyeglasses. Most magnifying lenses are made so that they're held at a specific distance from your face, but can be incorporated into the lens of a pair of prescription glasses and used for reading or detail work. However, the same power of the magnifier transposed to your glasses will require that you hold objects much closer to your eyes to be seen, which makes it more difficult to get proper lighting onto the object. The size of the lens correlates directly with magnifying strength: As a magnifying lens increases in size, its strength decreases. Conversely, the smaller the lens, the greater its power.

Stand and hand-held magnifying lenses: These magnifying lenses have a fixed focal distance, which can be helpful if you have difficulty holding objects at the correct distance for proper magnification. Hand-held magnifiers are placed flat against reading material and brought toward your eyes; stand magnifiers are placed on top of the material, which is read while seated. Both stand and hand-held magnifiers can be purchased with a battery or AC-powered light source built into the device.

Telescopic devices: These are special lenses that work like miniature telescopes. They can be mounted on a pair of eyeglasses to watch television or a movie; in some circumstances, they can also be used for driving. Telescopic devices improve clarity by making objects appear closer. Telescopic glasses with special filters or stand-mounted magnifiers containing a light source may help reduce glare and increase contrast (better distinction between light and dark).

Closed-circuit television: Personal reading devices, also called *closed-circuit televisions* (CCTV), use television cameras to read regular print, then blow it up on a monitor so that newspaper, magazine, or book type is three inches or more in size. Closed-circuit televisions now also come in portable personal versions. They can allow you, for example, to read product labels and prices when you're shopping. Or, they can be connected to desktop CCTV systems. Though many people with low vision find these machines helpful, they cost about $1,500 to $3,000 and may not be covered by Medicare or other health insurance.

With all optical aids, especially the CCTV, one should use as little magnification that allows the material to be read as possible in order to see enough of the word or words to provide continuity of thought. Too much magnification limits the field of words.

Nonoptical Low Vision Aids

Electronic auditory devices: Auditory devices use synthesized speech technology to verbalize information to the person using them. These include talking medical equipment, such as thermometers and blood pressure monitors, as well as watches and alarm clocks; talking Caller ID that announces the telephone numbers of those calling; talking numeric pagers; computer systems that render print into spoken language; and calculators that let the user rely on hearing rather than vision. Some devices can scan the text in a book or magazine then read the material aloud.

Spills and burns from hot liquids are a hazard for people with low vision, but there's even an ingenious device that senses—and beeps—when liquid comes too close to the rim of a cup. Among the other innovative products available are lighted tie racks and prescription bottle magnifiers that enlarge type on prescription medications.

Large-print products: Inexpensive, low-tech options include large-print versions of playing cards, kitchen timers, bingo cards, and bold-lined paper, as well as big-button television remote controls, clocks, and telephone pads. And, of course, many books and newspapers come in large-print versions. Listening to books on audiotape is another popular option.

EYE OPENER

If you have low vision, one of the most useful things you can do is to get closer to the object you're viewing. Contrary to popular belief, holding reading material near your eyes or sitting close to a television set won't harm your eyes. Your eyes adjust to the distance. Another simple solution is to correct your lighting by placing reading material closer to the light. To avoid glare, which can sometimes make seeing more difficult, opt for high-intensity halogen bulbs, which are available where light bulbs are sold. They will shine light directly on your reading material, not over your shoulder. The best position for a good light source with a solid, opaque shade is between your eyes and the reading material, in front of your face so that you avoid light and glare on your glasses and eyes.

THE FALLPROOF HOME

Low vision can increase your risk of falling, a major health hazard for older Americans. In the United States, one out of every three adults age sixty-five and older falls each year, making falls the leading cause of injury and deaths among people of that age. Besides visiting your eye doctor regularly to make sure your prescription is up to date, reduce your risk of falling or injury from falling by:

• Exercising regularly. Exercise improves strength, balance, and coordination, and can make you feel better. Before starting an exercise program, speak to your doctor.

• Making your home safer. Here are just a few ideas:
  – Remove tripping hazards, such as papers, books, boxes, clothes, and shoes from the stairs and other places where you frequently walk.
  – Reroute or cover up electrical cords on floors with a rug with rubber backing.
  – Use nonslip mats in the bathtub and on shower floors.
  – Install grab bars next to the toilet and in the tub or shower, and have handrails put in on both sides of all stairs.

— Put food and other kitchen items on the first shelf of cabinets where you can easily reach them without a stepstool.

— Clean up floor spills immediately.

— Replace old light bulbs and illuminate your home with brighter ones (be sure not to exceed the proper wattage recommended for each lamp). To reduce glare, use lampshades and frosted bulbs.

— Make sure your staircase is well lighted. Light switches should be at both the top and the bottom of the stairs. Your stairway light bulbs should provide enough light so that you can see each step and the top and bottom of landings.

— Put nonslip treads on all barewood steps.

— Remove loose area rugs from the bottom and top of stairs.

— Keep a lamp and flashlight near your bed to avoid fumbling in the dark.

— Put a slip-resistant rug next to the bathtub so that you can get in and out safely.

— In all rooms, arrange furniture so that there's a clear pathway between rooms and high-traffic areas.

— Install light switches at room entrances, so you don't have to navigate a darkened room to get to the light switch.

EYE OPENER

To fend off falls, get your hearing checked by your family doctor (who may refer you to a hearing specialist). Besides eyesight, hearing plays an important role in balance and space perception; poor hearing can increase your chances of falling. According to the

National Institutes of Health, about one-third of Americans between sixty-five and seventy-four and one-half those age eighty-five and older have hearing problems.

Getting Help for Low Vision

In addition to using various gadgets, those with low vision can learn a few simple, clever tactics to compensate for their diminished sight.

Ophthalmologists, optometrists, occupational therapists, and clinical social workers can all help with this effort. The overall strategy is to make the best use of your remaining vision. So, for example, if you have diminished contrast vision, rethink your choice of place setting: dark coffee is easier to see when poured into a white mug, and a fried egg is more easily seen when served on a black plate. A technique, for example, as simple as sorting and placing dollar bills in different sections of your wallet, or folding them according to different denominations, can help you distinguish your money. Marking steps and floors with contrasting paint, safety tape, or tread strips to highlight their edges can make them much more easy to see. You can also adapt your computer so that you can continue to do word processing, use spreadsheets, and perform other computer-related tasks.

To help you learn visual rehabilitation skills that teach you to manage your daily activities and maintain an independent lifestyle, you might consider seeking the services of vision-rehabilitation professionals. Therapists sometimes make home visits to recommend specific changes, such as rearranging furniture for easier maneuvering, labeling foods and medications with large print to make them easier to identify in the refrigerator or medicine cabinet, and positioning reading lamps so that they're shining directly on the page, to eliminate glare. Talk with your doctor or vision specialist about other rehabilitation methods that include ways to better navigate the outside world—bus stops, sidewalks, and street corners—with enhanced use of the other senses, as well as optical aids.

Don't go it alone. For more information on the education and rehabilitative services and agencies offered in your area that can provide you with strategies for best using your remaining vision *see* "Resources," on page 229.

EYE OPENER

Continuing or giving up driving is an important judgment call for those suffering from low vision. Don't make that decision until you or your family have all the facts and you've had a comprehensive eye exam, preferably done by a low-vision specialist. Depending on your state's visual requirements and your condition, you may be able to continue driving and maintain your independence if you use special equipment, such as miniature telescopes, called bioptics, *that are designed into a pair of eyeglasses to enhance peripheral vision (recommended for patients with impaired central-field vision). A warning—these telescopic driving glasses are controversial. They may allow one to pass the driver's test on a stationary eye chart, but are usually a major risk factor in driving. The central vision area is magnified and the surrounding vision is not.*

Summary

☛ Low vision can be caused by many conditions, the more common being cataract, glaucoma, diabetic retinopathy, optic nerve disease, AMD, or eye injury.

☛ Many aids and services are available to enhance low vision, so independence can be retained.

9

Safeguarding Your Sight

As you have learned, millions of Americans age forty and older are affected each year by glaucoma, cataracts, and age-related macular degeneration—three leading causes of blindness or impaired vision. One in six adults age forty-five and older has some sort of vision problem. The risk of developing a serious, potentially irreversible eye disorder increases with age.

According to Prevent Blindness America, twice as many Americans will be a victim of these serious eye conditions by the year 2030. With the graying of the population in the United States, it is estimated that the number of persons affected with age-related macular degeneration will grow from 2.4 million (1970 statistics) to 6.3 million in 2030, making it a leading public-health problem.

It doesn't have to happen. Although aging puts you at greater risk for these serious eye diseases and other eye problems, loss of sight doesn't necessarily go hand in hand with growing older. There's a lot you can do to preserve your vision—preventive measures can help protect you against devastating vision impairment. An estimated 40 to 50 percent of all blindness can be avoided or treated. In this chapter, we'll discuss practical sight-saving strategies you can try at home and at work to help you see clearly now and into the future.

Get Regular Checkups

Regular eye exams are the cornerstone of visual health as you age. We can't stress enough the importance of getting your eyes examined routinely to detect potentially blinding eye problems. For people ages forty to sixty-four without eye diseases or risk factors for disease, that means having an exam every two to four years by an optometrist or an ophthalmologist. If you're sixty-five or older, you should schedule an exam with an ophthalmologist every one to two years—even if you don't have noticeable symptoms. If you have a family history of eye disease or other risk factors, such as diabetes, glaucoma, or a previous eye injury, you may need to have your eyes examined more frequently. Speak to your eye doctor about a schedule that's right for you.

To detect unsuspected eye conditions, your eye doctor is your best friend. Frequently, only an exam can detect eye disease in its earliest, most treatable stages. Don't wait until your vision deteriorates, or until you notice blurring, redness, or pain to have an eye exam. One eye can often compensate for the other while an eye condition progresses, all the while stealing your sight. Regular screening by an eye doctor is a must.

Eat with Your Eyes in Mind

Besides getting regular eye exams, there is one very important thing you can do to protect your vision. Studies show that eating a nutritious diet, with lots of fruits and vegetables, promotes sound health and may boost your resistance to eye diseases, such as age-related cataracts and macular degeneration, as well as delay their onset and slow their progress over time.

More specifically, emerging research shows that a diet rich in foods that contain antioxidants may help maintain eye health, as well as your general health. *Antioxidants* are certain vitamins and other substances that combat *free radicals*. These unstable oxygen molecules may damage your body's cells and lay the foundation for disease if they're not neutralized by antioxidants.

How do antioxidants do their job? On a microscopic level, your body is a battleground against infection and disease, and oxygen—the very element everyone needs for survival—is both the good and bad guy. Each oxygen atom we breathe contains a pair of *electrons* (charged electrical particles). As you metabolize food and your body goes through its normal processes, however, some oxygen molecules shed one electron. They thus become *rogue* molecules, otherwise known as *free radicals*. Free radicals can attack healthy cells of all kinds, hoping to steal an electron to stabilize themselves. Free radicals can be neutralized by antioxidants, which may donate an electron to free radicals. If not neutralized, free radicals are thought to damage cell DNA, laying the groundwork for cancer, and a host of other equally formidable diseases, including two of the most common age-related eye conditions—cataracts and macular degeneration.

In macular degeneration, the light-sensitive macular cells in the retina break down, causing loss of the vision needed to see fine detail. Oxidative damage is thought to be the culprit, at least in part, because the retina is exposed to more oxygen than any other part of the body; the retina constantly uses oxygen to focus light. The macula is also loaded with polyunsaturated fatty acids, which are particularly prone to free-radical attack. Over the years, as the eye becomes less efficient at repairing oxidative damage from free radicals, lesions may form on the macula that cause it to degenerate.

With cataracts, the lens may cloud due to oxidative damage from exposure to the sun's harmful blue ultraviolet light, which is thought to produce free radicals that ultimately fog the lens. Antioxidants may help combat free-radical damage by absorbing blue ultraviolet light to hinder it from doing its damage.

Sight-Saving Superstars

Studies suggest that one particular category of antioxidants, called *carotenoids,* may play a role in maintaining your eye health, as well as enhancing your overall resistance to disease. *Carotenoids* are antioxidants that give fruits and vegetables their natural color—the red of a tomato, for example, on the green of broccoli. Two carotenoids in particular, lutein and zeaxanthin, which are related to the antioxidant beta-carotene, may be particularly beneficial in protecting eye health. (Both lutein and zeaxanthin are found in large quantities in the retina and in the lens.)

According to subsets of two major Harvard Medical

School studies—the Nurses' Health Study and the Health Professionals' Follow-up Study—in which 77,000 women and 36,000 men were monitored after twelve years, those who ate the most lutein and zeaxanthin had about a 20 percent lower risk of cataract surgery than those who ate the least. More specifically, women who ate spinach and other greens at least twice a week had an 18 percent lower risk than women who consumed the foods less than once a month. Men who ate broccoli more than twice a week had a 23 percent lower risk than men who consumed it less than once a month.

Although lutein and zeaxanthin may be responsible for protecting aging eyes, researchers are careful not to label them the answer. Something else yet undiscovered in green and other vegetables may protect eyes from disease.

Moreover, lutein and zeaxanthin aren't the only substances in food thought to potentially impact eye health. The groundbreaking Eye Disease Case-Control Study, which involved 876 participants, 356 of whom had advanced stages of age-related macular degeneration, showed that those who consumed more carotenoids in general (such as lycopene, the carotenoid in tomatoes) decreased the risk of age-related macular degeneration by 43 percent. Moreover, vitamin C (also an antioxidant) may be a contender. Studies of women in their fifties, sixties, and seventies have shown that those who consumed sizeable amounts of vitamin C had fewer cataracts. Other studies have also shown that nutrients such as vitamin E, selenium, folic acid, vitamin A (which converts to beta-carotene in the body), zinc, and *omega-3 fatty acids* (the heart-healthy fat found in fish and other foods) may also protect the eye from age-related disease.

In general, every fruit and vegetable is believed to have a different nutrient-protective profile. For the best health insurance for your eyes and the rest of your body, it's a good idea to cast a wide net and eat a variety of fruits and vegetables every day as part of a balanced diet.

More Reasons to Eat Your Five a Day

Currently, studies are underway to further investigate the association between long-term eye health and the consumption of lutein and zeaxanthin, as well as other nutrients. As a result, it's not yet possible to say definitely which nutrients best prevent age-related eye diseases, such as cataracts and macular degeneration, and what should be eaten by whom and in what quantities. Research does indicate that the odds are good that eating plenty of lutein and zeaxanthin-rich produce, especially green leafy vegetables, such as broccoli or spinach, will help. By consuming more of these foods, you may increase the density of these carotenoids in your eye's retina and lens, and protect them from harmful oxidative damage.

Diseaseproofing Your Diet

The National Cancer Institute recommends consuming five or more servings of fruits and vegetables a day to reduce your overall cancer risk. (Cancer, by the way, is considered an age-related disease, because its risk increases with age.) This amount of produce may well help reduce the risk of cataracts and macular degeneration as well, although more studies need to be done before firm recommendations can be made. In any event, according to United States Department of Agriculture (USDA) food consumption surveys, Americans age fifty-one and over get an average of only 3.85 servings of produce a day, which suggests that we're probably not eating enough produce to optimally protect our health. Moreover, the produce we consume isn't always in the healthiest form. According to food consumption surveys, the potato is the most popular vegetable in America, and 50 percent of the time it's in the form of french fries, which, of course, tend to be high in fat and relatively low in nutrients. According to the USDA, neither white nor sweet potatoes contain lutein or zeaxanthin, although they do contain other potentially eye-healthy nutrients, such as vitamin C and beta-carotene.

EYE OPENER

To get a cornucopia of lutein and zeaxanthin in your diet, as well as protect yourself from a host of other diseases, such as heart disease and cancer, it's generally a good idea to aim for five or more daily servings of fruits and vegetables. One serving equals one medium fruit or half cup of small or cut-up fruit; three-fourths cup of 100 percent fruit juice, one-fourth cup dried fruit, or one-fourth cup raw or cooked vegetables.

Getting plenty of lutein and zeaxanthin in your diet isn't difficult. These antioxidants can be found in a variety of fruits and vegetables, especially kale, spinach, turnip greens, collards, corn, Brussels sprouts, raw baby carrots, romaine lettuce, peas, green beans, persimmons, broccoli, and summer squash (zucchini); smaller amounts can be found in oranges and tangerines. Since all carotenoids are fat soluble, you may enhance their absorption by eating them with some fat, such as spinach sautéed with a drizzle of olive or canola oil, or a spinach salad with a side of vinaigrette dressing. Eggs are also a source of lutein/zeaxanthin, although they're no match for the produce mentioned.

EYE OPENER

If you're considering either changing your diet to include more foods rich in antioxidants and/or taking vitamin supplements, consult your doctor. You may have other health considerations that could be affected by these dietary changes.

FOCUS ON GETTING MORE PRODUCE

If you're like many Americans, you need to add at least two daily servings of produce to your diet to make your five-a-day quota, and reduce your risk of a variety of age-related diseases. To give your diet and your eyes the protective power of produce, here are several ways to work more fruits and vegetables into your diet.

• **Sneak in produce wherever you can.** At meals, sneak fruits and vegetables into the foods you already eat. For example, top off your morning cereal or yogurt with fruit, or and add it to homemade breads, cakes and cookies, salads, and sauces. Layer sandwiches with dark leafy greens such as spinach and watercress; order your burger or chicken or fish sandwich with extra lettuce, tomato, and onion. Roll bean sprouts, shredded cabbage and slices of green or red pepper into tortillas or flat bread; heap salsa onto low-fat tortilla chips; toss petite peas, tomatoes, onion, celery, carrots, and peppers into a salad. Smuggle mushrooms, peppers, zucchini, onions, and carrots into pasta sauce, meat loaf, soup, stew, and chili.

To make life interesting and more disease protective, go beyond the basics: apples, oranges, and bananas. Experiment with more exotic options, such as papayas, mangos, raspberries, blueberries, melons, cranberries, strawberries, and fresh pineapple. Tropical fruits and berries are especially potent sources of disease-fighting antioxidants.

• **Drink some veggies.** Vegetables contain antioxidants, as well as fiber and other vitamins and minerals that provide health insurance against a host of diseases—from cancer to high blood pressure to macular degeneration. Don't feel like doing all of that chopping? No matter. To get in more veggies, simply drink vegetable juice more often. It's a quick way to meet your produce quota. Moreover, most vegetable juices are blends, so they provide more unique combinations of vegetables you might not otherwise eat. Variety maximizes the kinds of disease-fighting nutrients you'll have on board. For example: V8 has the juice of tomato, carrots, celery, beets, parsley, lettuce, watercress, and spinach. Added bonus: Many vegetable juices today are calcium fortified (check the label), to also help you ward off bone-weakening osteoporosis, an important consideration as you get older.

• **Start your day with a double.** As a rule, the earlier in the day you start chipping away at your quota of five or more servings of fruits and vegetables a day, the easier it is to get those servings in. Begin your day with twelve ounces of juice, such as orange, grapefruit, or tomato (double the usual serving size), and you'll get two servings before you even leave the house.

• **Reorganize your refrigerator.** What we eat is often what we see first when we look in places where we store food. With this in mind, move sealed bags of baby carrots, precut red and green pepper strips, and broccoli florets to the top shelf instead of hiding them in the lowly crisper bin. (The same goes for fruit.) Slide a container of hummus, baba ghanoush (pulverized eggplant), nonfat salad dressing, or yogurt dip next to them. You'll be enticed as soon as you open the refrigerator door.

• **Choose fruit for dessert.** Dessert is a great place to add fruit to your diet. If you find fresh fruit too puritanical for your tastes, try fresh fruit sorbet. With less fat than frozen yogurt and only 100 calories per half cup, brands made with fruit juice (check the label) are a sweet way to get vitamin C. (By the way, tastes do change. If you opt for fresh fruit for dessert once a week or so, you may find yourself seeking it out more often.) If you're dying for something more traditionally sweet but still healthy, seek out fruit and vegetable delights such as reduced-fat carrot cake, chocolate zucchini cake, blueberry or apple pie, or pumpkin cheesecake (low fat, of course) at farm stands and bakeries.

Should You Take Eye Vites?

Scan the shelves of your local pharmacy and you're apt to see dozens of brands of eye vitamin supplements marketed commonly called *eye vites* for eye health, such as Ocuvite, Xangold, and Bright Eyes, some of which contain lutein, zeaxanthin, and vitamin C, and combinations of other nutrients. Although it may be tempting to think you can just pop a pill for good eye health—and research studies involving certain supplements, such as vitamin C, have shown them to be beneficial in preventing cataracts—you may be better off fortifying yourself with food and its formidable team of disease-fighting antioxidants, such as lutein and zeaxanthin, nutrients, and phytochemicals.

According to the National Eye Institute, there is currently little direct scientific evidence to support a claim that taking supplements containing lutein, for example, can decrease the risk of developing age-related macular degeneration or cataracts. In a twelve-year study involving over 73,000 women forty-five years of age or older, those who used multivitamins or separate supplements of vitamins C, E or A didn't decrease their risk of developing cataracts compared to those who didn't use them.

Moreover, vitamin pills may not convey the same disease-fighting benefits as whole foods over time. In fact, in some studies, megadoses have even increased disease risk. For example, in the 1980s, beta-carotene, another carotenoid, showed great promise in reducing the risk of cancer and heart disease. But large clinical trials of beta-carotene *supplements* showed that those supplements had little or no effect on heart disease, and actually increased the risk of lung cancer among smokers.

Nonetheless, if you're considering taking an eye vitamin, speak to your eye doctor for a recommendation. In the meantime, you may be advised by your family doctor to take a regular multivitamin to make sure your diet is nutrient dense. This is especially important as you get older, because it becomes harder for the body to make and use certain key nutrients. After age sixty, for example, the body begins to lose its ability to make vitamin D, which is essential for absorbing calcium to prevent bone-weakening osteoporosis, and to control blood pressure. As a result, it's even more important to get vitamin D from your diet or from a supplement, especially if you don't get much exposure to sunlight (sunlight helps your body produce vitamin D).

However, if you take an eye vitamin supplement in lieu of a regular multivitamin, you could be missing out on key nutrients you may need. If you take an eye vitamin in addition to your regular multivitamin, you may be getting too much of some nutrients, which can prove harmful. Mega amounts of vitamin C over the long haul, for example, can lead to gastric irritation and kidney stones. There's also growing evidence that supplements with over 100 percent of the recommended dietary allowance for vitamin A may be too high for people over age sixty, because the liver has become less efficient at clearing the vitamin from the body. Even folic acid, hailed for its ability to reduce the risk of heart disease, which is now being added to grain products such as bread and flour as part of the government food fortification program, can mask a vitamin B12 deficiency if overconsumed.

If you take a multivitamin as advised by your doctor, go ahead and stick with it. If your eye doctor advises you to take an eye vite, be sure to mention that you're already taking a multivitamin to avoid overconsuming nutrients. Also, try to fortify your diet with plenty of fruits and vegetables. Build your eating pattern on a variety of plant foods, including whole grains, fruits, and vegetables. For good general health, you should also choose some low-fat dairy products and low-fat foods from the meat and beans group each day.

HERBAL REMEDIES AND YOUR EYES

It's estimated that Americans spend over $2.5 billion a year on herbal remedies, such as St. John's wort, black cohosh, ginseng, and bilberry extract for various health conditions. And, they're not just sold in health food stores anymore. Your local pharmacy is likely to carry them, making them seem more official. As herbal remedies gain in popularity, there's something you should know: There's little to no scientific evidence in this country showing their efficacy, and the Food and Drug Administration does not regulate them. In essence, the natural remedies you're buying could be benign—or more powerful than prescription drugs. Moreover, herbal remedies have the potential to cause health or eye problems, especially if you exceed the recommended dosage, and take different supplements and/or prescription medication simultaneously. According to the American Optometric Association, black cohosh, for example, has been reported to cause clotting in the blood vessels in the back of the eye, and St. John's wort may enhance ultraviolet damage to the eye's crystalline lens.

Still, there are herbs that may present benefits to patients but present no known harm to the eyes. If you're considering taking any herbal remedy or if you're already taking an herbal remedy, tell your eye doctor. It's vital that your eye doctor be aware of this, especially if you're currently being treated for an eye disease, such as cataracts, glaucoma, or macular degeneration. Your eye doctor can advise you of any possible adverse interactions between herbals and prescription medications.

There Has Never Been a Better Time to Stop Smoking

Smoking is associated with all three major age-related eye diseases—glaucoma, age-related macular degeneration, and cataracts. According to a subset of the Physician's

Health Study I, a Harvard Medical School study involving nearly 21,000 U.S. male physicians spanning 13.6 years, researchers found a relationship between smoking and the development of cataracts. Although past smokers had a 23 percent less risk of cataracts when compared to current smokers, they still had a greater risk of cataracts than those who had never smoked. This study also showed that smoking-related damage to the eye's lens might be reversible if one stops smoking.

A subset of another major study, the Nurses' Health Study, which lasted twelve years and involved 31,843 registered nurses ages fifty to fifty-nine, showed that women who currently smoked twenty-five or more cigarettes a day had a two-and-one-half times increased risk of age-related macular degeneration than women who never smoked. Smokers who had smoked this amount but quit, had a relative risk of age-related macular degeneration of twofold.

Clearly, the more you smoke, the more you're at increased risk for age-related eye diseases. Certainly, you're better off if you never smoked in the first place, but that doesn't mean you can't benefit by quitting smoking now—no matter what your age or how long you've been lighting up.

In general, smoking is thought to cause hardening of the arteries that nourish the eye. It may also generate free radicals—those unstable oxygen molecules that may lead to cell changes that may jeopardize eye health, and do further damage by decreasing the level of antioxidants (compounds that neutralize free radicals) in the blood circulation, aqueous humor, and other eye tissue. Smoking is also a leading cause of lung, laryngeal, esophageal, oral, pancreatic, bladder, and cervical cancers, and heart disease. So, you'd be wise to quit smoking for a variety of health reasons. Many studies show that tobacco-related health effects decline substantially as time away from smoking increases; some of the benefits begin within just months after quitting.

GETTING HELP WITH KICKING THE HABIT

Statistics show that half of all smokers have quit, so you can, too. For help in quitting, ask your doctor about stop-smoking aids such as Zyban, a nonnicotine pill that affects the pleasure center in your brain to minimize withdrawal symptoms such as irritability, and nicotine-replacement therapies such as nicotine gum, the nicotine patch, or nicotine nasal spray. On average, studies show using these aids can double your chances of success. Combining any one of these products with smoking-cessation counseling—even as brief as talking for a few minutes about quitting with your doctor—quadruples your chances of quitting success. The more support you have, the better your chances of quitting for good. Stop-smoking programs are available at local hospitals and health centers. Call your local health department for programs in your area.

According to the Centers for Disease Control and Prevention's Office on Smoking and Health, here are several other important steps you should take that can help you kick the habit.

• **Don't think you can just smoke fewer or safer cigarettes.** Even a few cigarettes a day can be harmful to your health, even if they're lower in tar and nicotine. The only safe choice is to quit smoking altogether.

• **Write down why you want to quit.** If improving your health isn't motivating you to quit, find another good reason. Stopping smoking is tough. To quit, you must be motivated.

• **Set a quit date.** A firm date in mind will help establish your psychological commitment to quitting.

• **Rid your home, car, and workplace** of all cigarettes and ashtrays; it's one of the most fundamental ways to help you avoid temptation.

• **Once you've quit, quit.** Don't back down and tell yourself you can have just a puff. That's enough to get you hooked again.

EYE OPENER

With the opening of cigar bars across the country, and celebrities wielding cigars on magazine covers, cigar smoking has increased dramatically since 1993 among men and women, according to the National Cancer Institute. Cigars are often perceived as a healthier alternative to cigarettes. But don't kid yourself.

When it comes to smoking tobacco products, there's no safe version. Even smoking a cigar as little as once a month is accepting some amount of health risk as opposed to not smoking at all. Cigars may be just as dangerous to your health—and your eyes—as cigarettes. Compared to cigarette smokers, cigar smokers tend to smoke fewer cigars. However, because a cigar is bigger than a cigarette, containing more tobacco, a cigar smoker smokes longer, so the period over which you're exposed to the carbon monoxide, tar, and carcinogens is longer.

And, because cigar smokers hold the toxin-filled smoke in their mouth and upper throat, they're at increased risk of cancer of the oral cavities or the esophagus than cigarette smokers but, like cigarette smokers, they can also put themselves at risk for lung cancer. Many cigar smokers, particularly if they also smoke cigarettes, have a tendency to puff on a cigar and then draw the smoke deep into their lungs. They get the worst of both worlds. Overall, the harmful effects of cigar smoke are a dose-response relationship, meaning the more you smoke, the more damage you do to your body. Among consistent cigar users, one cigar is equivalent to four cigarettes.

The healthful benefits of not smoking cigars far outweigh the trendy pleasure they may provide. If you don't smoke cigars, don't start. If you smoke cigars, quit. If you're addicted, speak to your doctor. Like quitting cigarette smoking, there are effective nicotine replacement therapies available for quitting smoking, including nicotine gum, the patch, spray, and an inhaler, as well as individual and group counseling.

Invest in the Right Sunglasses

Throughout *The Aging Eye*, we've mentioned the importance of wearing sunglasses to protect your eyes from sun-related eye damage. After all, sunglasses aren't just fun to wear.

They're necessary to safeguard your sight. Researchers have established a link between eye health and eye disease, particularly cataracts and macular degeneration, and long-term exposure to the sun's harmful ultraviolet (UV) radiation. Sunglasses are essential to block the sun's UV light from damaging your delicate eye tissue.

EYE OPENER

Eye damage from the sun is cumulative. Your eye retains the sun damage you got as a child. Still, it's never too late to wear your shades.

Although you've probably heard plenty about UVA and UVB rays, UV light actually has three wavelengths:

☞ *UVA* is long, looks almost blue in the visible spectrum, and is responsible for skin tanning and aging.
☞ *UVB* is shorter, more active, and linked to sunburn and skin cancer (a large portion is absorbed by the atmosphere's ozone layer).
☞ *UVC* is short and completely absorbed by the ozone layer.

All told, UVA and UVB rays, which are invisible, can be especially harmful to your eyes, causing cataracts and age-related macular degeneration. They may also contribute to benign growths on the eye's surface, cancer of the eyelids and skin around the eyes, and snow blindness, a temporary but painful sunburn on the eye's surface.

The easiest way to protect your eyes from the sun's hazardous radiation is to wear a wide-brimmed hat or cap and UV-absorbing eyewear. A hat or cap will block roughly 50 percent of the UV radiation, and will reduce the UV rays that may enter the eyes from above or around glasses. Sunglasses that filter 99 to 100 percent of the sun's UVA and UVB rays can help reduce your risk of eye damage tremendously. Sunglasses are labeled according to guidelines for UV protection established by the American National Standards Institute (ANSI). There are three categories:

☛ **Cosmetic:** lightly tinted, good for daily wear. Blocks 70 percent of UVB rays, 20 percent of UVA, and 60 percent of visible light.

☛ **General purpose:** medium to dark lenses, fine for most outdoor recreation (most glasses fall into this category). Blocks 95 percent of UVB, 60 percent of UVA, and 60 to 90 percent of visible light.

☛ **Special purpose:** Extremely dark, with UV blockers, recommended for very bright conditions such as beaches and ski slopes. Blocks 99 percent of UVB, 60 percent of UVA, and 97 percent of visible light.

In general, it's best to simply select sunglasses with the ANSI label that filter 99 to 100 percent of the sun's UVA and UVB rays to help reduce your risk of age-related eye damage. Look for sunglasses that specify "filters 99 percent" or "filters 100 percent" of the sun's ultraviolet radiation on the label. Labels that merely claim "provides UV protection" don't cut it; be sure the percentage of the UV rays blocked is specified. Just because a lens appears dark, doesn't mean it's able to block out UV radiation. In fact, dark sunglasses without UV protection can fool your eyes and actually do more damage than no sunglasses at all. Under these conditions, your eyes are particularly vulnerable to sun damage because your pupils dilate from the darkness; meanwhile, the sun's UV rays stream in.

Keep in mind that sunglasses needn't bear a designer label or cost hundreds of dollars to do their job properly; even inexpensive sunglasses can be effective, as long as they have the ANSI label and filter 99 to 100 percent of UV rays. (You can also get regular eyeglasses with clear UV protection. Ask your eye doctor.)

In terms of what color sunglass lenses to buy, there's some evidence that blue light from the sun precipitates age-related macular degeneration, and lenses with a red, amber, or orange tint may provide better protection against this light. You may find less distortion, however, with gray, green or brown, lenses. If you aren't sure what kind of sunglasses to buy, consult an eye-care professional.

Play It Safe

Whether or not you've been diagnosed with an eye disease, it's important to protect the vision you have from eye injuries. Injuring your eye puts you at increased risk for glaucoma, cataract, and retinal detachment caused by trauma. Emergency rooms across the country treat 40,000 sports eye injuries annually. Whatever your sport, whatever your age, you need to protect your eyes. If you participate in rugged recreational sports, such as snow skiing, racquetball and basketball—the leading cause of eye damage in twenty-five to sixty-four-year-olds—it's important to wear protective eyewear with polycarbonate lenses to safeguard the remaining sight you have. Polycarbonate is a shatterproof, lightweight plastic that can protect your eyes from potentially damaging debris, such as a wayward volleyball or other airborne objects. (Regular eyeglasses don't provide adequate protection for high-risk sports. In fact, because they're not shatterproof, they may even increase your risk of eye injury.) If you have vision in only one eye, or limited vision in one eye, it is very important always to wear polycarbonate lenses during your waking hours.

EYE OPENER

If you participate in sports in which there's a lot of reflected sun, such as boating, water, or snow skiing, consider wraparound frames with polarizing lenses, which can protect the skin surrounding your eyes, and reduce glare tremendously.

Before buying protective polycarbonate eyewear, check the label to be sure it's certified by the American Society of Testing Materials or the Protective Eyewear Certification Council. (If you're buying glasses from an optician or a sales representative at a sporting goods store, ask if the frame and lenses meet these standards.) Otherwise, the glasses may not be able to withstand the impact of balls, elbows, ski poles, and tree branches. Protective eyewear is also available by prescription. Ideally, it's best to have a pair of protective eyeglasses fitted by your eye doctor. Protective eyewear shouldn't distort vision, and should provide good peripheral vision and protection, and fit comfortably. Prescription-free protective eyewear is also available for contact-lens wearers.

EYE OPENER

If you have only one eye functioning properly, be sure to wear protective eyewear at all times to protect the vision in your good eye.

Protect Your Eyes Around Your Home

It's also important to wear protective eyewear when you're working around your home. According to Prevent Blindness America, household products cause more than 32,000 serious eye injuries each year. Wear protective eyewear any time, for example, when you're hammering nails, mowing the lawn, or using the snow blower. Without adequate polycarbonate protective eyewear, nails can flip into the eye; rocks and other debris can ricochet off the curb or the house. (For outdoor chores, don't count on regular shop goggles to do the job; they're not shatterproof and may increase your risk of eye injury.)

When you're working with chemicals such as drain and oven cleaner, wear splash goggles (available at hardware stores). Also be sure to read all manufacturer's instructions and warning labels on products before using them, and avoid mixing different types of cleaning agents. If you do get chemicals in your eyes, irrigate your eyes immediately. Put your eyes under cold running water from the faucet or the shower. If you're in a remote location and water isn't available, you can flush out chemicals with most any beverage—surprisingly, even iced tea, cola, or orange juice will do.

If you cut or puncture your eye, bandage it lightly without pressure, and see your eye doctor immediately. If you receive a blow to your eye, lightly apply a cold compress to reduce pain and swelling, and seek emergency care promptly.

Enhance Your Night Vision

As you get older, you may notice that you have more trouble seeing well at night. It may be more difficult, for example, to make out street signs and the dividing lines on the highway; the glare from oncoming headlights may bother you, and in general, it may take your eyes longer to adjust to darkness. Although poor night vision can be a symptom of conditions such as cataract, glaucoma, and diabetic retinopathy, most everyone's night vision naturally diminishes to some extent as they get older. From age twenty to sixty, it's estimated that the average eye's ability to distinguish contrast declines two-and-one-half times, and continues to gradually decline.

The reason night vision becomes more difficult to manage than when you were younger is that as the lens of the eye ages, it naturally thickens and becomes less transparent and more opaque. As a result, some of the light that should go to the retina, where it connects to the optic nerve, gets scattered to other areas of your eye. Scattered light reduces contrasts, similar to what happens if you try to see a movie in a theater with the lights on. Scattered light can also cause painful glare and cause colors to blur.

As soon as you notice reduced night vision, see your eye doctor for an exam; this is an important step to rule out cataracts, diabetic retinopathy, and other medical conditions. Meanwhile, depending on your eyes' reaction to darkness, your doctor may recommend a different eyewear prescription for night driving if you wear glasses or contacts. You can also have antireflective coating applied to your lenses, which reduces glare from lights at night. You can also improve your night vision by doing the following:

☞ Avoid looking directly at oncoming headlights when you're driving at night. To reduce glare, look to the right of the road and slightly downward instead.

☞ Be sure your eyeglasses, windshield, mirrors, headlights, and taillights are clean before setting out.

☞ Don't forget about your car's high-beam lights. Use them as often as you can when night driving.

☞ Stay on well-lit roads, and use your low beams for fog and rain.

☞ Drive more slowly if necessary for safety.

☞ Avoid wearing tinted glasses or sunglasses when you drive at night, but wear sunglasses with UV protection during the day; daytime sunglass wearing can help your eyes better maintain normal night vision.

EYE OPENER

If seeing at night becomes especially difficult, your safest bet may be to get a ride from a family member or a friend, take public transportation, or simply take your car trips only during the day.

Guard Against Computer Eye Strain

Spending many hours in front of a television or computer screen, or working in poor light doesn't do medical harm, but these types of activities or conditions can tire or strain the eyes, and ultimately their owner. Eyestrain occurs when the muscles that move your eyeball become fatigued from constantly being used in one position for a long period. It's equivalent to running all day without taking a break. Frequent computer users are also known to experience symptoms such as headaches, blurred vision, eye irritation, double vision, pain in the eyes, excessive blinking or squinting, and excessive tears or dry eyes.

If your eyes are already dry due to dry eye syndrome, it is apt to worsen if you often do computer work. Symptoms may be caused by poor lighting, glare, an improper work station setup, vision problems of which you may not be aware, or simply because you're not blinking enough. In normal situations, we tend to blink about twelve to fifteen times per minute. However, when we're reading or concentrating, we tend to blink less often. This can dry the eyes. When you blink, the upper lid comes down and picks up tears from the bottom like a windshield wiper, bringing them across your eye. Blinking allows the eye to rest for a short time as it cleans and rewets the eye surface to maintain clear vision.

Besides dry eyes and eyestrain, frequent computer users often experience neck, shoulder, and back pain because they're holding their head at an odd angle; their glasses may not be designed for computer work, or they may be bending toward the screen because their vision needs to be corrected. Either posture can cause muscle spasms or pain in the neck, shoulders, and back.

Whether you're using your computer at work or simply using it at home to correspond via e-mail or browse the Internet, be sure to see your eye doctor for a thorough eye exam if you spend more than a few hours at a computer each day. If your eyes hurt, you may need to have your prescription checked. In some cases, you may be prescribed single-vision, multifocal, or special computer glasses. Several lenses are made specifically for computer users. Most are no-line multifocals that have a wide area for viewing the computer in the upper portion of the lens, and an area in the lower portion for close work, such as looking at the keyboard. Because they don't correct distance vision as well as lenses for general wear, they're limited to use at the computer. Special computer contact lenses may also be an option to correct the situation. Intermediate-distance glasses may provide adequate vision for computer and desk work, depending on monitor–eye distance.

Meanwhile, there are also several simple ways to reduce your risk of muscle fatigue and give your eyes a rest.

☞ If you tend to get absorbed in your work, take frequent breaks. Every few minutes, look past your computer or out the window for a few seconds, to give your eyes a break from looking in one position for a long time. Also, every twenty to thirty minutes, get up and take a walk. Moving around every so often boosts circulation, and gives all your muscles a chance to rejuvenate. (Better yet, do some deskercises, such as those that follow on page 187.) If you have software with a timer, set it to go off to remind yourself to move. Or, paste a Post-it note on your computer monitor as a health break reminder. The same holds true when you're doing any close work, such as reading, paperwork, distance vision, or sewing.

☞ If your eyes are dry or itchy, use an over-the-counter lubricating eye drop (artificial tears) periodically. Products without preservatives, or those with *disappearing preservatives,* which break down when they come in contact with the eye, tend to be the least irritating. Your eye doctor can suggest the best brand for you.

☞ To reduce glare on your computer screen, reposition lamps and adjust blinds or drapes when necessary; invest in a glare-reduction micromesh screen for your computer. Don't face your computer screen toward the window. Your monitor should be at a right angle to all natural light sources.

☞ Clean your screen often with a clean, damp cloth.

☞ Choose a light screen with dark letters; it's easier on the eyes than a dark screen with light letters.

☛ Adjust your screen so that it's four to nine inches below eye level, and twenty to twenty-six inches from your eyes.

☛ Fix your form. What you're after is a neutral desk posture, one that puts little pressure on your back, neck, and shoulder muscles, and prevents you from straining to see the screen. To sit properly and maximize your computer comfort:

1. Sit squarely and firmly against the backrest of your chair. You should be able to place two fingers behind your calves. If you don't have this clearance, put a lumbar support pillow (available at retail computer stores) against the backrest of your chair. Your feet should also be firmly grounded. If they don't touch the floor, get a foot rest, or use a thick book, such as a telephone directory.

2. Place your monitor and keyboard so that they're directly in front of you, not off to one side. Place reference material as close to your screen as possible, with the screen and holder at the same distance from your eyes. Data in a copy holder should be right next to your monitor. Neck twisting is a no-no.

3. Position your keyboard so that it's flat or tilting downward, with your computer mouse at the same height. Ideally, the angle at your elbow should be greater than ninety degrees and your wrists should be flat. If this isn't possible because your desk is too high, consider getting a pull-out keyboard tray (also available at retail computer stores) to allow your arms to be lower than desk level.

4. Sit an arm's length away from your monitor to avoid eyestrain and subsequent neck craning. When positioned properly, you should barely be able to graze the front of your screen with your hand.

DESKERCISES ANYONE CAN DO

To stay loose and relaxed at work and help keep muscle strain at bay, practice the following exercises.

- **Shoulder shrug:** Tilt your head toward your right shoulder and shrug this shoulder at the same time. With your head still tilted, drop your shoulder, then raise it again. Repeat on the left.
- **Shoulder straddle:** Press your right shoulder forward and turn your head toward it. At the same time, press your left shoulder back. Repeat on the other side.
- **Winging it:** Sitting or standing, raise your elbows so that your forearms run perpendicular to your body. Slowly press your shoulderblades together.
- **Stirring dough:** Circle your hand in front of you as if you were stirring dough. Repeat on the other side.
- **Push and pull:** With both arms stretched in front of you and palms facing outward, gently push your hands forward while pulling your shoulders back. Do this exercise at three heights—near your ears, in the middle of your body, and near your thighs.

Moreover, exercise regularly, if you can. Strength training, especially, will develop more muscle mass and muscle tone as well as boost the oxygen to muscles, which can help increase resilience to computer-related muscle fatigue.

Defend Your Eyes Against Diabetes-Related Disease

Diabetes mellitus is one of the oldest diseases known to man; it can affect the eyes and the nervous system, as well as the heart, kidneys, and other organs. In the twenty-first century, diabetes is becoming one of the most prevalent diseases. Simply put, diabetes is a condition in which the body is unable to adequately break down glucose, the simple carbohydrate your body depends on for fuel. Over the last forty years, as the nature of the American population has changed, the rate of diabetes has more than tripled. A larger senior population, an increase in obesity, and more people from high-risk ethnic backgrounds have resulted in the current statistics: sixteen million Americans with diabetes, and 650,000 new cases diagnosed each year.

EYE OPENER

Today, as in ancient times, there is no cure for diabetes. Thanks to advances in medical research, it's no longer the frightening condition it once was. With proper management, a person with diabetes can live a full and active life.

There are two basic types of diabetes. *Type 1,* insulin-dependent diabetes, is an inherited disorder in which the body doesn't produce any insulin, a hormone meant to control glucose levels that helps get food energy to your cells. About 10 percent of people with diabetes have this form of the disease, which is usually first diagnosed in children or young adults. Having a parent or other close relative with the disease puts you at increased risk for type 1.

Roughly 95 percent of the 16 million Americans with diabetes have *type 2,* the form of diabetes that results from the body's inability to make enough, or properly use, insulin. Those with type 2 diabetes have abnormally high levels of glucose circulating in their blood.

Like type 1, type 2 diabetes, also called *adult-onset diabetes,* has a genetic component. African-Americans, Native-Americans, Hispanics, and people of Asian ancestry are more at risk than Caucasians. According to the American Diabetes Association, a person can inherit a tendency to get type 2 diabetes. It usually takes another factor, such as obesity, to bring on the disease. Being at an unhealthy weight is, by far, the greatest risk factor for type 2 diabetes. It's estimated that more than 80 percent of those with type 2 diabetes are overweight. Moreover, the risk of developing type 2 diabetes more than doubles with every 20 percent increase over an individual's ideal body weight.

If you have diabetes—either type 1 or type 2, you're at greater risk for health problems like heart disease, stroke, kidney disease, and even death. You're also at increased risk for diabetic eye diseases, such as glaucoma, optic neuropathy, and cataracts. In fact, those with diabetes are almost twice as likely to develop glaucoma and cataracts than those who don't. You're also more likely to suffer from vision loss from the effects of a chronic condition called *diabetic retinopathy*—damage to the blood vessels of the retina. According to the American Academy of Ophthalmology, diabetic retinopathy is the leading cause of blindness in working-age American adults.

When diabetic retinopathy first begins, called the *nonproliferative* stage, small blood vessels in your eye that nourish your eye's retina, may swell, forming pouches of blood. These damaged blood vessels may leak fat and protein that are deposited on the retina in patches. The blood vessels may also bleed into the retina and the vitreous. You may not notice any change in your vision at this mild stage of the disease unless you develop a condition called *macular edema.*

Macular edema may cause retinal blood vessels of the eye to leak blood or other fluid into the macula—the part of the retina that allows you to see fine details—to swell and blur vision. It may then become difficult to read and do other close work. If your eye doctor suspects that you have macular edema, you may be asked to undergo a diagnostic test called *fluorescein angiograpy,* which can help your doctor find leaking blood vessels in your eye. During this test, your doctor will inject a special dye into your arm. Photos are taken as the dye makes its way through blood vessels in your retina. During the proliferative stage, treatment isn't always necessary, especially if you don't have symptoms, but you should get your eyes checked at least once a year to make sure it's not getting worse.

After several years, if the disease progresses to the *proliferative* stage, blood vessels in your eye eventually become damaged and shut down; fragile new blood vessels grow in the surface of the retina. These blood vessels can break and bleed into the vitreous, the clear, jellylike substance that fills the center of your eye. As the vitreous becomes clouded with blood, light can't pass through the eye to the retina. As a result, you may experience blurred or distorted vision. Scar tissue can also form from these new blood vessels, which can pull the retina away from the choroid, causing retinal detachment, which can lead to blindness if not promptly treated. (For more information on retinal detachment, see page 140.)

EYE OPENER

Because of the potential complications, those with diabetes are twenty-five times more likely to become blind than those without the disease, which is why it's so important to keep close tabs on the condition.

Detecting Retinopathy

Besides dilating your pupils, your eye doctor will perform a *visual acuity test* (to measure how well you see at distances) and *tonometry* (to measure fluid pressure in the eye) and take a close look at your retina with an *ophthalmoscope*. If the retina examination detects the hemorrhages and exudates that characterize diabetic retinopathy, other tests might be done.

If you have diabetes or a family history of the disease, don't put off getting your eyes checked at least once a year. (Don't hesitate to see your eye doctor more frequently if you notice any changes in your vision or if you already have eye disease.) Studies show that many people with diabetes don't get an annual dilated-eye examination. Diabetic retinopathy and other diabetic eye diseases can progress without symptoms. While they're stealing your sight, you may not notice any changes in your vision.

Treating Diabetic Retinopathy

Fortunately, there are several treatments available for diabetic retinopathy. According to the National Eye Institute, you have a 90 percent chance of keeping your vision even if you have advanced retinopathy if you get treatment before your retina is severely damaged.

☛ **Scatter photocoagulation:** In this outpatient procedure, also called *panretinal photocoagulation,* your eye doctor will dilate your pupil and numb your eye with eyedrops, then use a special laser to make hundreds of tiny burns on your retina. These burns shrink abnormal blood vessels, stopping them from growing and leaking into the vitreous, or causing the retina to detach. The purpose of scatter coagulation is to stabilize vision, not necessarily restore it. During the procedure, you may see flashes of light and feel a slight stinging sensation. You'll need someone to accompany you home. You should also wear sunglasses since your pupils will remain dilated. Side effects may include temporary blurred vision or loss of peripheral vision.

☛ **Focal photocoagulation:** Your eye doctor will aim a high-energy laser directly at leaking blood vessels in the macula to prevent blurry vision from getting worse. Unlike scatter photocoagulation, light is focused on a single spot.

With either scatter or focal photocoagulation, you may need more than one treatment to preserve your vision.

☞ **Vitrectomy:** If your retina has detached, or a significant amount of blood has leaked into your eye, your eye doctor may opt for a *vitrectomy*, a surgical procedure discussed earlier, that's often done under local anesthesia, which removes the vitreous humor through aspiration and replaces it with saline solution. You won't notice any difference between the saline solution and normal vitreous. After the operation, which may be inpatient or outpatient, your eye will be red and sensitive. You may need to wear an eye patch for a few days to protect your eye, and apply eyedrops for several days to prevent infection and inflammation. For more information on vitrectomy, see page 145.

EYE OPENER

When someone is diagnosed with diabetes, a doctor's first prescription is usually for lifestyle changes. Typically, it will call for weight reduction, a better diet, and a hefty dose of exercise. In fact, between 10 percent and 20 percent of those with type 2 diabetes will be able to control diabetes through these measures and not need to take medications or injections.

Taking Care of Your Eyes When You Have Diabetes

If you've been diagnosed with diabetes, it's important to

keep your blood glucose levels as close to normal as possible by following the treatment plan recommended by your doctor. The longer you have diabetes, the more apt you are to develop retinopathy. According to Prevent Blindness America, more than 40 percent of those who have diabetes for fifteen years or more have some blood vessel damage. Some of these people go on to suffer from the most serious result of the disease: severe vision loss or blindness.

Controlling your diabetes doesn't insure against diabetic retinopathy, but tight control of your diabetes and your blood sugar can delay and possibly prevent diabetic retinopathy from developing and/or progressing to blindness. According to the Diabetes Control and Complications Trial, a major nine-year clinical trial involving 1,441 volunteers with insulin-dependent diabetes, the group who tried to keep their blood sugar levels under tight control— as close to normal as possible—had much less eye, kidney, and nerve disease. In those who already had retinopathy, the condition progressed only half as often. In general, keeping your diabetes under tight control means:

☛ Following your meal plan carefully.
☛ Taking your insulin or diabetes medication as prescribed.
☛ Exercising regularly.
☛ Testing your blood sugar as recommended by your doctor.
☛ Recording your blood-sugar values in a diary and reviewing them with your doctor.
☛ Watching for any symptoms of complications, such as blurry vision.
☛ If you take insulin, ask your doctor if and when you

should check your urine for *ketones,* an unhealthy compound found in urine that signifies your diabetes is uncontrolled. It's especially important to check for ketones if you've been sick or unable to follow your meal plan.

Besides working to control your blood sugar, if you have diabetes, you should see your eye doctor at least once a year for a comprehensive eye exam that includes dilating the pupils with eyedrops so that your doctor can closely examine the back of your eye. An eye exam allows the eye doctor to check your retina for unusual blood-vessel changes, such as leaking, swelling, or pale, fatty deposits on the retina, or damaged nerve tissue.

A LIFETIME PLAN FOR PREVENTING TYPE 2 DIABETES

If you're at risk for type 2 diabetes, start working now to prevent its development. You're at increased risk for type 2 diabetes if you have a close family member (sibling or parent) with the disease, are overweight or don't exercise regularly, have a triglyceride level above 200 and low HDL (good) cholesterol or have high blood pressure. You're also at high risk for type 2 diabetes if you are Native-American, Latino or African-American, or were diagnosed with gestational diabetes or delivered a large baby (nine pounds or more). Getting older also raises the risk: Between 10 percent and 15 percent of the population over age 60 has the disease. Your risk also rises if you've ever had elevated blood glucose.

Fortunately, there's a lot you can do to prevent or at least delay the onset of type 2, and reduce complications from the condition if you are diagnosed.

- **Maintain a healthy weight:** Avoiding weight gain will help maximize your body's responsiveness to insulin. Many people who develop type 2 diabetes are overweight. Gaining weight, especially in your abdomen, increases the body's demand for insulin. Early on, beta cells in the pancreas may pump out extra insulin to keep up with the increased blood-sugar demands. Over time, however, those beta cells become deficient and lose the ability to make extra insulin.

When that happens, *glucose* (sugar) builds up in the blood. High blood sugar damages the eyes, the nervous system, the kidneys, and the heart. If you keep your weight down, you won't stress your pancreas as much. Even if you have diabetes and are overweight, shedding just ten to fifteen pounds can improve your symptoms and may prevent some complications.

- **Get active:** Regular exercise can help reduce your risk of diabetes, not only by keeping your weight in check but by helping your body become more efficient at using glucose. (See your doctor before starting an exercise program.) Exercise takes some glucose out of the blood to use for energy during and after exercise, which lowers blood glucose levels. As a result, your pancreas doesn't have to work as hard, so it will, presumably, last longer. (For the same reason, if you already have type 2 diabetes, physical activity can help you manage the condition.) Moreover, exercise, especially heart-pumping activity, such as walking, bicycling, or jogging, can also help prevent heart disease, the leading killer of people with diabetes.

- **Eat a balanced diet:** To minimize your risk of type 2 diabetes, eat meals that are high in low-fat complex carbohydrates, such as fruits, vegetables, and whole grains, like whole-wheat bread, oatmeal, and rice. A balanced diet that includes plenty of these kinds of foods makes it easier to maintain a healthy weight; it can also help moderate blood glucose levels and can help reduce your risk of complications, such as diabetic retinopathy.

- **Get tested regularly:** If you're at risk for type 2 diabetes, talk to your doctor about getting tested. (If you're not certain if you're at risk for diabetes, take the Diabetes Risk Test at the American Diabetes Web site at www.diabetes.org.) Don't wait for your doctor to bring it up. Evidence suggests that physicians tend to ignore the risk factors and not discuss them with patients. Meanwhile, if type 2 diabetes goes undetected, serious complications, such as diabetic retinopathy, can set in.

A fasting blood glucose test, a simple blood test that's the preferred diabetes diagnostic test, gauges the amount of glucose in your blood (126 mg/dl or more indicates full-blown diabetes). Under some circumstances, your doctor may advise you to also have a glucose-tolerance test, which involves drinking glucose and having blood drawn at specified intervals. If you're at increased risk for type 2 diabetes, your doctor will probably advise you to get tested yearly. Because the risk of diabetes increases in everyone with age, you should have a fasting blood glucose test every three years if you're over age forty-five.

DIABETES: WHAT TO WATCH FOR

If you experience any of the other signs of diabetes described here, or are at increased risk for diabetes because of risk factors, such as your ethnic background or a family history of diabetes, see your doctor and get tested regularly. To preserve your sight, it's important to get the condition under control as soon as possible.

- blurred vision
- excessive thirst
- increased frequency or volume of urination
- unexplained weight loss (sometimes accompanied by increased appetite)
- weakness, fatigue, and nausea
- slow healing of cuts and wounds
- intense itching

Protect Yourself from Diseases Associated with Vision Problems

In addition to diabetes, several other chronic diseases can threaten the health of your eyes. Being diagnosed with any one of these conditions is another good reason to see your eye doctor regularly.

Atherosclerosis: You may be familiar with this term in relation to the arteries of the heart. However, *atherosclerosis*—blood vessels clogged with cholesterol and other fatty deposits—can occur in the blood vessels of the retina as well. When retinal blood vessels become completely blocked, retinal cells become deprived of oxygen and nutrients, a situation that can lead to temporary or permanent blindness. If you experience blurred vision or blindness in one or both eyes, see your eye doctor immediately.

Stroke: Sudden blindness in one or both eyes and/or blurred vision can also be warning signs of a stroke, the condition in which a blood vessel to the brain becomes blocked, impeding blood flow and depriving the brain of oxygen and nutrients. Stroke is the third leading cause of death in the United States, and most common among older people; your chances of having a stroke more than doubles for each decade after age fifty-five. In addition to vision changes, other signs of a stroke include sudden numbness or weakness in your face, arm or leg, especially on one side of the body; sudden confusion, trouble speaking or understanding; sudden trouble walking; dizziness; loss of balance or coordination; and/or sudden severe headache with no known cause. If you experience one or more of these symptoms, or know of someone experiencing them, even for just a few minutes, call 911, or get to the hospital right away. A stroke is a life-threatening emergency.

To reduce your risk of stroke, avoid smoking and work to control your blood pressure. If you drink, do so in moderation (that is, no more than one drink a day for women, two drinks a day for men); maintain a healthy weight and exercise regularly. If you have heart disease, follow your doctor's instructions for controlling the condition. People with heart disease have more than double the risk of stroke of those whose hearts are healthy.

Hypertension: Years of *hypertension,* also known as high blood pressure, defined as 140/90 or higher, can speed the normal aging of blood vessels in the eyes, causing blurred vision. In severe cases, blood vessels in the retina can rupture, a situation that requires immediate treatment. Moreover, high blood pressure can lead to heart disease, the leading cause of death for both men and women in the United States. Often called *the silent killer,* high blood pressure may be symptomless until it's too late. Your best defense: Get your blood pressure checked regularly. High blood pressure can often be controlled through lifestyle changes, such as following a low-fat diet that includes plenty of fruits, vegetables, and fat-free and low-fat dairy products; avoiding high-sodium foods, such as many processed and convenience foods; drinking only in moderation, if at all; and maintaining a healthy weight. Your doctor may also prescribe medication to control your blood pressure, especially if lifestyle changes don't lower it enough. To protect your eyes and your health, be sure to follow your hypertension treatment plan.

Rheumatoid arthritis: If you've been diagnosed with rheumatoid arthritis, a disease in which the body's immune system forms antibodies that attack healthy tissues (in this case, in the joints, hands, and feet) instead of serving its normal protective function, you're at increased risk for Sjögren's syndrome. This chronic condition affects between one and four million Americans, many of whom are women between the ages of forty-five and fifty-five. Sjögren's syndrome occurs when the body's immune system mistakenly attacks moisture-producing glands, including tear glands, causing eye inflammation or eyes that become so dry, they often burn or feel gritty. Rheumatoid arthritis and Sjögren's syndrome can lead to eye inflammations or

damage to the cornea. Your eye doctor can prescribe eyedrops applied several times daily that can alleviate uncomfortable dry eyes associated with the condition. Inflammation within the eye from the arthritis may call for more
aggressive medications.

Lupus: In about seven percent of people with this particular
autoimmune disease, which causes episodes of inflamed
joints, tendons, and other connective tissues and organs,
white puffy patches appear on the retina, due to insufficient
blood supply. Although the patches don't affect vision, they
can be detected during an eye exam and can be a sign of damage to the retina or a symptom that other organs of the body
aren't receiving the proper amount of blood.

Graves' disease: A condition in which the thyroid gland
produces too much of the hormone thyroxine; in some
cases the muscles of the eyeball that control movement and
the orbital fluid swell and cause the eyeball to bulge forward. This is called exophthalmus. In these cases, the optic
nerve can become compressed, threatening vision. With
Graves' disease, the eyelids can also retract, exposing the
cornea to injury or dryness. Early symptoms of Graves' disease include irritated eyes, double vision, excessive tearing
or dry eyes, or sensitivity to light. The exophthalmus may
limit eye movement, causing double vision. In rare cases,
vision loss may result. Fortunately, treatment for Graves' disease is available. Eyedrops can help relieve eye irritation as
can cool compresses and sunglasses. In more serious cases,
in which the optic nerve becomes compressed, your doctor
may prescribe corticosteroids or even surgery.

COMMON EYE MYTHS DISPELLED

Adopting better eye-care habits can improve your chances of protecting your eyesight for a lifetime. However, eyesight myths lurk everywhere. From the misguided advice you get from a friend to the latest information on the Internet, it's easy to fall prey to bad eye-care information. Are your eyes as healthy as they could be? Take this true-or-false quiz to check your eye-care knowhow.

1. Doing eye exercises will put off the need for glasses.
False: Eye exercises may strengthen muscles within the eye, but they won't improve or preserve your vision.

2. Reading in dim light will worsen your vision.
Not exactly. Although dim lighting won't adversely affect your eyesight or harm your eyes, it will tire your eyes more quickly. The best way to position a reading light is to have it shine directly onto the page. If the light shines over your shoulder, it's likely to cause a glare.

3. It's best *not* to wear glasses all the time. Taking a break from glasses allows your eyes to rest.
False. If you need glasses for distance or reading, use them. Attempting to read without reading glasses will simply strain your eyes and tire them. Using your eyes or wearing your corrective lenses for long periods day after day won't worsen your vision or lead to any eye disease.

4. Eating carrots is good for the eyes.
There is some truth in this one. Carrots, which contain vitamin A, are one of several vegetables that are good for the eyes. Fresh fruits and dark green, leafy vegetables, which contain more antioxidants, such as lutein and zeaxanthin, may be even better. (Raw carrots are a modest source of

lutein/zeaxanthin.) Antioxidants may help protect the eyes against age-related cataracts and macular degeneration. Eating any vegetable or supplement containing these vitamins or substances won't prevent or correct basic vision problems, such as nearsightedness or farsightedness. Too much vitamin A can actually harm your eyes and health.

5. Staring at a computer screen all day is bad for the eyes.
True. Although using a computer won't permanently harm your eyes, looking at a computer screen for long periods will contribute to *eyestrain,* another term for tired eyes. Adjust lighting so that it doesn't create a glare or harsh reflection on the screen. Also, when working on a computer or doing other close work, such as reading or needlepoint, it's a good idea to rest your eyes briefly every hour or so to lessen eye fatigue.

6. Getting an eye exam is only really necessary if you're having problems.
False. Everyone should have a proper eye exam regularly, even if they're not having any noticeable symptoms. For good measure, have your eyes examined every two to four years by an optometrist or ophthalmologist if you're between forty and sixty-four, and every one to two years by an ophthalmologist after age sixty-five. In addition, see an ophthalmologist if you experience any of the following symptoms or problems: bulging of the eyes; a change in the color of the iris; crossed eyes; a dark spot in the center of your field of vision; difficulty focusing on near or distant objects; double vision; dry eyes with itching or burning; excess discharge or tearing; eye pain; floaters or flashes; haloes (colored circles around lights); hazy or blurred vision; loss of peripheral vision; redness on or around the eye; spots in your field of vision; straight lines appearing wavy or crooked; sudden loss of vision; trouble adjusting to dark rooms; unusual sensitivity to light or glare, and/or a veil blocking your vision.

GETTING FINANCIAL HELP FOR EYE CARE

If you need financial assistance to treat any eye problem, contact the social-work department at your local hospital; they may be aware of community resources that are available to help those who are facing financial and medical problems. Your health-insurance plan and/or Medicare may pay all or a portion of the cost. In addition, *see* "Resources," page 229 for a comprehensive list of organizations that provide financial aid to individuals for eye care. If you are over sixty-five, a United States citizen, and have not had a medical eye exam for three years, call 1-800-222-EYES for a referral to an ophthalmologist who will care for your eyes for a year at no out-of-pocket expense, as part of The National Eye Care Project of the Foundation of the American Academy of Ophthalmology.

Consider Participating in Age-Related Eye Disease Clinical Trials

If you've been diagnosed with eye disease, you may be interested in participating in a clinical trial. Clinical trials are often the best hope for people faced with serious diseases. If you participate in a clinical trial, you can expect the highest-quality medical care and a considerable amount of medical attention for the treatment of your condition. The only sure way to determine whether a new treatment is safe, effective, and better than other treatments is to try it on patients in a clinical trial. In cases in which eye diseases run in families, your participation may lead to better care for your family members. If more patients enrolled in clinical trials, more safe and effective drugs might be available much sooner than they are now.

What Is a Clinical Trial?

A *clinical trial* is a carefully designed study that closely monitors the progress of a patient as he proceeds through treatment with a new drug, device, or medical therapy that's not yet on the market or otherwise available. Clinical trials are sponsored by government agencies, such as the National Eye Institute of the National Institutes of Health; pharmaceutical companies; health-care institutions, such as health maintenance organizations; and organizations that develop medical devices or equipment. Your don't necessarily need to travel to a major university or teaching hospital to participate in a clinical trial. They're usually conducted through a network of study sites across the United States, including medical centers, hospitals, universities, and doctors' offices.

Before a drug, device, or medical treatment can be tested in humans, it must undergo extensive testing in the laboratory and be the subject of animal studies. Only after these tests are conducted and show promising results, can the treatment enter a phase I clinical trial. During *phase I,* the main questions researchers are asking is: Can this drug be given? Does it work? Researchers test a new drug or treatment on a small group of people for the first time to evaluate its safety and appropriate dosage. If results prove promising, the treatment enters into a *phase II* clinical trial, during which more people receive the treatment, and safety and effectiveness is again evaluated to test whether the drug, in fact, works.

If phase II testing is clearly positive, the treatment is evaluated in a *phase III* clinical trial with even more patients to confirm its effectiveness, monitor side effects, and compare it to standard therapy. It also provides a clearer picture of the percentage of patients for whom the drug is safe and effective, and its side-effect profile. After all these clinical trials have been conducted, the results are submitted to the Food and Drug Administration, which then decides whether the drug or therapy should be approved for patients nationwide.

During an eye-related clinical trial, you will be randomly assigned to receive an experimental drug or treatment, or receive a standard treatment for the disease or a *placebo* (an inactive pill, liquid, or powder that has no treatment value). All clinical trials involve risks, as well as possible benefits. The treatment you receive may cause side effects, and there's always the possibility that a new treatment may not work any better than the standard treatment, or may be harmful. Some clinical trials involve more tests and doctor visits than you would normally undertake for your illness or condition. You will be expected to have eye exams and other tests. You may also need to take medications and/or undergo surgery. During a clinical trial, you will be carefully monitored throughout your treatment. Monitoring is performed both at the site at which you're being treated, as well as centrally, in the organization that's sponsoring the trial. This extensive monitoring helps ensure that patients receive the appropriate dose, have the treatment adjusted based on side effects encountered, and stay within the set clinical trial protocol. In addition, audits of records are performed to assure that the sponsoring organization and the doctors administering the treatment are abiding by the protocol. The government has strict guidelines and safeguards to protect people who choose to participate in clinical trials. Every clinical trial in the United States must be approved and monitored by the Institutional Review Board (IRB), which involves committees of professional and laypeople, including members who have no affiliation with the site performing the trial. The IRB makes sure the risks are as low as possible, and are worth any potential benefits.

Only patients that meet certain criteria may participate in a clinical trial. All clinical trials have guidelines or protocols as to which patients can participate. Guidelines are based on such factors as age, disease, medical history, and past and current treatment. Doctors and researchers evaluate patients based on these criteria and, if patients qualify, they may enter into a particular clinical trial.

If you're selected to participate in a clinical trial, you can quit at any time for no reason. Clinical-trial treatment isn't covered by all health plans; check your policy. However, the costs to the patient are usually taken care of by the clinical-trial program. To participate in an eye-disease-related clinical trial, ask your eye doctor about related clinical trials that are recruiting members for your condition. If your eye doctor isn't aware of any eye-related clinical trials for which you might be eligible, he or she can find out by calling The National Eye Institute Clinical Director's Office at (301) 496-6932. (Don't call directly; only your doctor should call on your behalf. She should have your medical records handy so that she can easily determine whether you qualify for the clinical trials.) You can also find out about clinical trials that are currently recruiting patients by logging onto the following web sites: www.nei.nih.gov, the web site for the National Eye Institute; www.clinicaltrials.gov, the web site for the federal government, which lists ongoing clinical trials; or www.centerwatch.com, a site that lists a wealth of information about clinical trials, including those pertaining to vision.

Summary:

☞ Although aging increases the risk of serious eye disease, vision loss doesn't have to go hand in hand with growing older.

☞ There's a lot that can be done to preserve vision including: getting regular eye exams; eating a balanced low-fat diet that contains plenty of produce; not smoking; and protecting your eyes from the sun, hazards around the home, and from other diseases, such as diabetes and other chronic conditions that can affect your eyesight.

☞ After diagnosis, consider participating in an eye-disease clinical trial. With your participation, you can expect the highest-quality medical care and attention. Your participation may also lead to the development of new drugs and therapies that can help treat you as well as others with your condition.

☛ Visit your eye doctor for regular checkups. It's the most important thing you can do to take good care of your eyes as you get older.

Appendices

Drugs Used to Treat Glaucoma
Drugs Used to Treat Dry Eye Syndrome

Appendix I.

Drugs Used to Treat Glaucoma

ADRENERGICS (TOPICAL)

Generic Name	Brand Name	Use	Side Effects	Comments
dipivefrin hydrocholoride	Propine	Reduces pressure, may dilate pupil briefly	Headache, stinging, redness, burning, transient blurring of vision	May cause pounding heart and fast heartbeat in some people

ALPHA-2 AGONISTS (TOPICAL)

Generic Name	Brand Name	Use	Side Effects	Comments
brimonidine tartrate	Alphagan	Lowers pressure by reducing fluid secretion and increasing outflow	Stinging, burning, redness of eyes, dry mouth, blurred vision, fatigue	Minimal effect on lungs and cardiovascular system

BETA BLOCKERS (TOPICAL)

Generic Name	Brand Name	Use	Side Effects	Comments
betaxolol	Betoptic, Betoptic S	Lowers pressure in eye by reducing production of aqueous humor	Stinging, irritation, blurred vision, tearing, allergic reaction	Elderly people are especially prone to side effects; may cause breathing problems for people with asthma; can slow heart rate for those with heart disease; may cause sense of mental and physical lethargy; men may experience a decrease in libido
carteolol	Ocupress			
levobunolol	Betagan			
metipranolol	OptiPranolol			
timolol maleate	Timoptic XE, Timoptic			

CARBONIC ANYHYDRASE INHIBITORS (ORAL AND TOPICAL)

Generic Name	Brand Name	Use	Side Effects	Comments
acetazolamide	Dazamide, Diamox (oral)	Lowers pressure, slows fluid production in the eye	Dizziness, diarrhea, loss of appetite, metallic taste in mouth, numbness or tingling in hands and feet, weight loss, fatigue, excessive urination, anemia, kidney stones, mental lethargy	Can lead to loss of potassium; eat potassium-rich foods, such as bananas and citrus fruit
dichlorphenamide	Daranide (oral)			
methazolamide	Neptazane (oral)			
dorzolamide hydrochloride	Trusopt (drops)		Burning, stinging, bitter taste in mouth, corneal inflammation, allergy	Also available in oral form. Drops have fewer side effects for most people
brinzolamide	azopt (drops)			Not available in oral form

MIOTICS (TOPICAL)

Generic Name	Brand Name	Use	Side Effects	Comments
carbachol	Isopto Carbachol, Miostat	Causes pupils to contract; lowers pressure by improving the outflow of drainage	Eye pain, stinging, blurred vision, change in near or distance vision, reduced night vision	May worsen other eye conditions, such as cataract; may cause breathing problems for people with asthma; may be associated with retinal detachment in people prone to the disorder
echothiophate iodide	Phospholine Iodide		Blurred vision, change in near or distance vision, reduced night vision, headache, eyelid twitching, tearing, sweating, diarrhea, cataracts	
pilocarpine	Adsorbocarpine, Pilagan, Pilocar, Pilopine HS		Blurred vision, change in near or distance vision, reduced night vision	

PROSTAGLANDINS AND DERIVATIVES (TOPICAL)

Generic Name	Brand Name	Use	Side Effects	Comments
latanoprost	Xalatan	Increases drainage of fluid through uveoscleral pathway	Burning, stinging, itching, redness, blurred vision	Used only once a day; some people report change in eye color due to increase in brown pigment in the iris; may make lashes grow longer
travoprost unoprostone bimatoprost	Travatan Rescular Lumagan	Unknown drainage of fluid through uveoscleral pathway		

Appendix II.

Drugs Used to Treat Dry Eye Syndrome

OPHTHALMIC LUBRICANTS

Generic Name	Brand Name	Use	Side Effects	Comments
hydroxypropyl methylcellulose	GenTeal Lubricant Gel	Relieves dryness and prevents further irritation by adding lubrication	Allergic reaction	
white petrolatum, liquid lanolin, and mineral oil	AKWA Tears, Duratears Naturale			

ARTIFICIAL TEARS

Generic Name	Brand Name	Use	Side Effects	Comments
carboxymethyl cellulose	Refresh Plus, Celluvisc, Theratears	Relieves dryness by adding moisture and lubrication	Allergic reaction	No preservatives
glycerin	Dry Eye Therapy		Allergic reaction	
hydroxypropyl cellulose	Lacrisert		Blurred vision, redness, sensitivity to light, stickiness of eyelids, allergic reaction	Some people may be allergic to preservatives; insert is placed in eye and dissolves
hydroxypropyl methylcellulose	Isopto Tears, Lacril, Moisture Drops, Hypotears			Drops; some people may be allergic to preservatives or the medicine itself
polyvinyl alcohol	AKWA Tears, Dry Eyes Lubricant, Just Tears, Liquifilm Tears		Allergic reaction	

Glossary

ACCOMMODATION The eye's ability to change the shape of the lens to bring close objects into focus.

AFTER-CATARACT An opacity that develops in the lens capsule after a cataract has been removed.

AGE-RELATED MACULAR DEGENERATION (AMD) A condition that causes loss of central vision due to the breakdown of cells in the macula. AMD is the leading cause of irreversible blindness in the United States and other industrialized countries.

AMD (DRY) This common type of age-related macular degeneration (AMD), which occurs in 90 percent of reported cases of AMD, causes small yellow spots, called *drusen,* or pigment deposits accumulation at the macula.

AMD (WET) This type of AMD, which affects 10 percent of all cases of AMD, causes abnormal blood vessels to grow in or beneath the retina, allowing fluid to seep into the tissue, damaging the macula, possibly causing blindness.

AMSLER GRID A pattern resembling graph paper with a dot in the middle, used to test for age-related macular degeneration;

AMD may be present if the lines near the spot look wavy.

ANTERIOR CHAMBER The space behind the cornea and in front of the iris; it's filled with aqueous humor.

ANTIOXIDANTS Vitamins and other substances that protect cells against oxidative damage from free radicals. Antioxidants are found in many foods; some are produced in the human body. Antioxidants include carotenoids and flavonoids.

AQUEOUS HUMOR The waterlike fluid that nourishes the eye, and fills the anterior and posterior chambers of the eye.

ASTIGMATISM A refractive error characterized by irregular curvature of the cornea or lens, causing distorted images.

ATHEROSCLEROSIS A condition in which blood vessels become clogged with cholesterol and other fatty deposits; the disorder can occur in the blood vessels of the retina, as well as in other blood vessels of the body. When blood vessels of the retina become completely blocked, retinal cells become deprived of oxygen and nutrients, a situation that can lead to temporary or permanent blindness.

BETA BLOCKERS These topical eyedrops, similar to beta blockers used to treat some types of heart disease, are commonly prescribed for glaucoma. Topical beta blockers lower pressure in the eye by reducing the amount of aqueous humor produced by the eye's ciliary body, which is just behind the iris.

BIFOCAL CONTACT LENSES These contact lenses have two corrective powers on one lens, one for distance and one for near vision. Like bifocal eyeglasses, they are available in lined or *progressive* (no line) form, in which there's no obvious separation between the two prescriptions.

BIFOCALS Corrective lenses that contain two prescriptions—an upper lens that corrects nearsightedness (for distance vision) and a lower lens that corrects farsightedness (for close vision).

Bifocals come in two styles, those with a visible horizontal line and those with a line that's ground so that it doesn't show. *Progressive,* or lineless, bifocals change gradually from distant correction at eye level to reading correction at the bottom.

BINOCULAR VISION   The ability of the two eyes to combine separate images into a single perceived image.

BLEPHAROPLASTY   Reconstructive eyelid surgery that removes excess tissue and restores vision to correct *ptosis* (drooping upper eyelids). This surgery, which usually leaves nearly invisible scars, tightens muscles and lifts the lid. It can be performed under local or general anesthetic on an outpatient basis.

CATARACT   A clouding or fogging of the eye's crystalline lens.

CHOROID   A thin membrane in the middle layer of the eye between the sclera and retina; replete with blood vessels, it supplies nutrients to eye tissue, including the rods and cones of the retina.

CILIARY BODY   A structure behind the iris comprised of muscles and blood vessels; its surface cells produce aqueous humor, and the ciliary muscles change the shape of the lens.

CLINICAL TRIAL   A carefully designed research study that closely monitors the progress of a patient as he proceeds through treatment with a new drug, device, or medical therapy that's not yet on the market or otherwise available to patients. Clinical trials are sponsored by government agencies; pharmaceutical companies; hospitals; health-care institutions, such as health maintenance organizations; and organizations that develop medical devices or equipment.

CONES   Specialized cells in the retina that are sensitive to color and light; they are most active in daylight, provide sharp vision, and are abundant in the macular area.

CONJUNCTIVA   The transparent membrane that lines the eyelid and covers the front portion of the sclera.

CORNEA The curved, transparent tissue that makes up the front of the eye, and through which light first passes.

CRYOTHERAPY Using cold or freezing temperatures to treat disease; it's sometimes used to control glaucoma or repair the retina.

CRYSTALLINE LENS A flexible, transparent globular body directly behind the iris that focuses rays of light onto the retina.

CUPPING An indentation in the optic disk that often occurs in glaucoma.

CYSTOID MACULAR EDEMA A cystic swelling of tissue in the macula that is sometimes a complication of cataract removal, other intraocular surgery, or inflammation.

DIABETES (TYPE 1) Also called *insulin-dependent diabetes,* type 1 diabetes is an inherited disorder in which the body doesn't produce enough insulin, a hormone to control glucose levels in the body.

DIABETES (TYPE 2) Also called *adult-onset diabetes,* this form of diabetes results from the body's inability to make enough, or properly use, insulin.

DIABETIC RETINOPATHY A potentially blinding complication of diabetes that damages tiny blood vessels in the eye's retina. As the disease progresses, fragile new blood vessels form in the retina and in the vitreous. Without timely treatment, these new blood vessels can bleed, cloud vision, and destroy the retina. Blindness can result. Diabetic retinopathy affects half of all Americans diagnosed with diabetes.

DRUSEN Tiny yellow deposits that form beneath the macula, and may be an indication of early stages of age-related macular degeneration.

DRY EYE A common, irritating syndrome usually caused by a decrease in tear production.

ECTROPION A tendency of the eyelids, more commonly the lower lid, to turn away from the eye.

ENTROPION The movement of the lid margin inward, toward the eye; more common in the lower lid.

EXCIMER LASER An ultraviolet laser used in refractive surgery to remove tissue from the cornea.

EXTRACAPSULAR CATARACT SURGERY A method of cataract removal by incision to extract the front portion of the lens capsule and the lens nucleus; the posterior capsule is left intact.

EXTRAOCULAR MUSCLES Six external, paired muscles that extend from the sides of the eyeball, behind the conjunctival wall, and from the back of the orbit; they direct the eye's circular, side-to-side, and up-and-down movements.

FILTERING PROCEDURE Conventional knife surgery sometimes used to treat glaucoma; it involves creating a new channel under the conjunctiva to improve the drainage of aqueous humor from the eye's anterior chamber.

FLOATERS Tiny clusters of protein or cells that drift through the vitreous humor and appear as black specks across the visual field. Although they're most commonly benign, they may precede retinal complications.

FLUORESCEIN ANGIOGRAPHY A diagnostic test that photographs blood vessels in the retina after the intravenous injection of a special dye.

FOCAL PHOTOCOAGULATION To perform this treatment, an eye doctor will aim a high-energy laser directly at leaking blood vessels in the macula to prevent blurry vision from getting worse. Unlike scatter photocoagulation, light is focused on a single spot. With either scatter or focal photocoagulation, more than one treatment may be needed to preserve vision.

FOVEA A pitlike depression in the middle of the macula.

FREE RADICALS Unstable oxygen molecules circulating in the body as a result of metabolism and other processes. Free radicals can attack healthy cells of all kinds, hoping to steal an electron from an atom in the cell to stabilize themselves. If free radicals aren't neutralized by antioxidants, which may donate an electron, they're thought to damage cell DNA, laying the groundwork for cancer and other equally formidable diseases, including age-related cataracts and macular degeneration.

FUNDUS PHOTOGRAPHY Diagnostic imaging that provides two- or three-dimensional pictures of the rear area of the eyeball, including the retina, optic disk, and retinal blood vessels.

GLAUCOMA A disease of the eye characterized by increased intraocular pressure.

GONIOSCOPY A diagnostic procedure employing a contact lens with prisms that permits inspection of the anterior drainage angle of the eye; used to detect glaucoma.

GRAVES' DISEASE A condition in which the thyroid gland produces too much of the hormone thyroxine. As a result, muscles of the eyeball that control movement swell and push the eyeball forward; in some cases, the optic nerve can become compressed, threatening vision.

HYPEROPIA An optical error in which light rays reach the retina before converging at a focus point; commonly known as *farsightedness*.

HYPERTENSION Also known as *high blood pressure*, this condition, defined as blood pressure that's measured at 140/90 or higher, can speed the normal aging of blood vessels in the eyes, causing blurred vision. In severe cases, blood vessels in the retina can rupture, requiring immediate treatment.

INTRACAPSULAR SURGERY A type of cataract extraction that removes the entire lens and its surrounding capsule.

INTRAOCULAR LENS IMPLANT A small plastic lens permanently fixed inside the eye to replace the natural lens after cataract extraction.

IRIDECTOMY A surgical procedure that removes part of the iris; may be performed on angle-closure glaucoma patients to facilitate the drainage of fluid from the eye.

IRIDOTOMY A surgical procedure that creates, usually by using a laser, a small opening in the outer edge of the iris; may be performed on closed-angle glaucoma patients to facilitate the drainage of fluid from the eye.

IRIS The colored ring of tissue in front of the lens that controls the size of the pupil and the amount of light that enters the eye.

LACRIMAL GLAND The gland that produces tears; located in the upper, outer section of the eye's orbit.

LASER An acronym for Light Amplification by Stimulated Emission of Radiation. A concentrated beam of light that emits intense heat or light energy at close range; its ability to be focused on a small area through optically clear tissue makes it useful in the treatment of several ocular diseases.

LASER IRIDOTOMY An opening in the iris created by laser to treat angle-closure glaucoma.

LASER PHOTOCOAGULATION The use of a laser to alter tissue, such as sealing off leaking blood vessels of the retina in age-related macular degeneration.

LASIK The acronym for Laser-Assisted In Situ Keratomileusis. During LASIK surgery, a flap is cut in the cornea with a *microkeratome* (microknife). Pulses from a computer-controlled laser vaporize some of the cornea's midsection to reshape it before the flap is replaced.

LENSOMETER A device used to determine the optical prescription of eyeglasses.

LIMBUS The junction between the transparent cornea and the sclera that serves as the site of the incision in various cataract and glaucoma operations.

LUPUS ERYTHEMATOSIS An autoimmune disease that causes episodes of inflamed joints, tendons, and other connective tissues and organs. In this disorder, white puffy patches can appear on the retina due to insufficient blood supply, signaling retinal damage and/or insufficient blood supply to other organs of the body.

MACULA The area of the retina packed with cones; responsible for acute, central vision.

MIOTIC A type of eyedrop that constricts the pupil; used to treat glaucoma.

MODIFIED MONOVISION This corrective eyewear option for the treatment of presbyopia uses a bifocal contact lens in one eye and a contact prescribed for distance in the other eye. The theory is that one has both eyes clear for distance and one eye for reading.

MONOVISION CONTACT LENSES An option for correcting presbyopia, especially relevant for those who wish to avoid eyeglasses. One wears a contact lens to correct near vision in one eye and, if necessary, a lens for correcting distance vision in the other eye. The eye that's set for close vision will be slightly blurred for distance.

MYDRIATIC A drug that dilates the pupil.

MYOPIA An optical error in which light rays meet and focus before reaching the retina; also known as *nearsightedness.*

OPHTHALMOLOGIST A medical doctor who specializes in medical and surgical eye disease.

OPHTHALMOSCOPE An instrument with lights and mirrors for examining the deep interior of the eye.

OPTIC DISK The head or front surface of the optic nerve, where all the retinal nerve fibers coalesce to carry the retinal image to the brain; corresponds with the blind spot.

OPTIC NERVE Resembling a cable, it emanates from the back of the eye and consists of specialized nerve fibers that transmit visual impulses to the brain.

OPTICIAN A technician who makes, fits, and delivers eyeglasses, contact lenses, or other optical devices that have been prescribed by an ophthalmologist or optometrist.

OPTOMETRIST A doctor of optometry who specializes in vision problems, as well as the diagnosis and limited treatment of eye disease.

ORBIT The bony socket that surrounds the eyeball.

PERIPHERAL VISION Side vision, or what the eye perceives outside the direct line of vision.

PHACOEMULSIFICATION A method of cataract removal that uses ultrasound waves to break up the lens so that it can be suctioned out with a needle; a small incision method of extracapsular cataract extraction.

PHOTOPSIA A sensation of sparks or flashes of light across the visual field.

PHOTOREFRACTIVE KERATECTOMY (PRK) A technique to improve myopia in which a laser reshapes the cornea. The procedure involves removing the surface layer of the cornea by gently scraping, and using a computer-controlled laser to reshape the *stroma* (the thick middle layer of cells in the cornea).

PNEUMATIC RETINOPEXY A technique for repairing retinal detachment, in which a bubble of special gas is injected into the eye during surgery. The gas pushes against the area of the retinal tear to block fluid from passing and promote adhesion to close the retinal hole and allow for retinal reattachment.

POSTERIOR CHAMBER The area behind the iris and in front of the lens; filled with aqueous humor.

PRESBYOPIA   The natural loss of the eye's ability to focus on close objects; noticeable in one's forties and progressing until the early sixties. It can be corrected with reading glasses.

PTOSIS   A drooping of the eyelid attributed to flaccid muscles.

PUPIL   The dark, circular hole in the middle of the iris.

REFRACTION   The deflection of light as it passes through one medium to another of different density; also refers to the measurement of the eyes to determine optical errors and prescriptions for correction.

RETINA   The innermost layer of the eye that converts light energy to electrical energy. Lining nearly three-quarters of the back of the eye, it consists of specialized cells that send visual images to the brain via the connecting optic nerve.

RETINAL DETACHMENT   A condition in which the retina separates from the choroid.

RODS   Light-sensitive cells, mainly in the peripheral retina, that respond best to darkness and dim light.

SCATTER PHOTOCOAGULATION   An outpatient procedure to treat retinal detachment, also called *panretinal photocoagulation,* in which a special laser is used to make hundreds of tiny burns on the retina. These burns shrink abnormal blood vessels, stopping them from growing and leaking into the vitreous or causing the retina to detach. Its aim is to stabilize vision, not necessarily restore it.

SCHLEMM'S CANAL   A circular drainage system located where the clear cornea, white sclera, and colored iris meet to form an angle.

SCLERA   The tough, protective coating of collagen and elastic tissue, seen as the white of the eye.

SCLERAL BUCKLING   A surgical technique that indents the sclera and choroid to reattach the retina; used to repair retinal detachments.

SJÖGREN'S SYNDROME   A condition in which the body's immune system mistakenly attacks moisture-producing glands, including tear glands, causing eye inflammation or eyes that become so dry that they often burn or feel gritty. Sjögren's syndrome can lead to eye infections or damage to the cornea.

SLIT LAMP (BIOMICROSCOPE)   An instrument that illuminates and magnifies external and internal structures of the eye, with the aid of a slit beam of light.

SNELLEN CHART   The standard eye chart used to test visual acuity.

STROKE   The condition in which a blood vessel to the brain bleeds or becomes blocked, impeding blood flow and depriving the brain of oxygen and nutrients. Sudden blindness in one or both eyes and/or blurred vision can also be warning signs of a stroke, the third leading cause of death in the United States.

TONOGRAPHY   A diagnostic test for glaucoma that evaluates the efficiency of the eye's fluid drainage system.

TONOMETRY   A glaucoma test that measures intraocular pressure.

TRABECULAR MESHWORK   A system of fine meshlike tissue in the anterior chamber, through which aqueous humor drains; located in the angle where the clear cornea, white sclera, and colored iris join.

TRABECULECTOMY   A standard surgical procedure for glaucoma that creates a new channel for fluid drainage from the anterior chamber to the subconjunctival space.

TRABECULOPLASTY   A laser procedure that burns small areas on the eye's trabecular meshwork to facilitate the flow of aqueous humor from the eye.

TRIFOCALS   Trifocal corrective eyewear contains three lenses— an upper lens to correct nearsightedness, a lower lens to correct farsightedness, and a small middle section lens located just above the bifocal segment on the lower part of the eyeglass lens to make corrections for middle-distance vision, such as when looking at a computer screen.

VISUAL ACUITY   The eye's ability to see sharply, usually measured in comparison to what a normal eye would see from twenty feet.

VISUAL FIELD   The scope of what the eye sees; includes central and peripheral vision.

VISUDYNE THERAPY   This FDA-approved therapy for the treatment of wet AMD is a two-step process in which the drug Visudyne, is injected into the body and arm, and is subsequently activated by shining a cool laser light into the eye.

VITRECTOMY   A surgical procedure that removes the vitreous humor through *aspiration* (suction) and replaces it with saline solution.

VITREOUS HUMOR   The transparent colorless mass of gel that lies behind the lens and in front of the retina, and fills the center of the eyeball.

YAG CAPSULOTOMY   A laser technique that creates a hole in the membrane opacity that forms in after-cataract; the opening allows light to enter clearly focused onto the retina.

ZEAXANTHIN   A carotenoid found in fruits and vegetables that may play a role in maintaining eye health, as well as overall health.

ZONULES   Thin gelatinous ligaments that attach the lens to the ciliary body and support the lens centrally behind the pupil.

Resources

Books

Cataracts: From Diagnosis to Recovery—The Complete Guide for Patients and Families
Julius Shulman, M.D.
St. Martin's Press, 1995, $11.95
A comprehensive guide to cataracts—from how cataracts form to what to expect in the recovery stage postsurgery.

Coping with Glaucoma
Edith Marks and Rita Mountauredes
Avery Publishing Group, 1997, $13.95
Highlights both conventional and alternative medications and procedures used to treat and diagnose glaucoma.

The Eye Book: A Complete Guide to Eye Disorders and Health
Gary H. Cassel, M.D., Michael D. Billig, O.D., and Harry G. Randall, H.D.

Johns Hopkins University Press, 1998, $18.95

A thorough, clearly written overview of eye care, that covers the prevention, detection, diagnosis, and treatment of eye problems, with a special focus on the changes and conditions that come with age.

Glaucoma: A Patient's Guide to the Disease
Graham E. Trope
University of Toronto Press, 1997, $8.95

A detailed look at glaucoma, from symptoms to diagnosis and treatment.

Macular Degeneration: The Complete Guide to Saving and Maximizing Your Sight
Lylas G. Mogk, M.D. and Marja Mogk
Ballantine Books, 1999, $13.95

Cowritten by a freelance writer and her mother, a practicing ophthalmologist who cares for a father with advanced macular degeneration, this book combines factual information about macular degeneration with firsthand tips on day-to-day living and personal insight into the stresses faced by those with vision loss and the people who care for them.

Making Life More Livable: A Practical Guide to Over 1,000 Products and Resources for Living Well in the Mature Years
Ellen Lederman
AFB Press, 1994, $19.95

Shows how to make simple adaptations in your home and environment for greater visibility, including furniture rearrangement, lighting, color and contrasts, use of appliances, and other safety precautions. Available in large print.

Vision-Related Organizations

The following organizations can provide resource information on eye care and disease prevention for patients and their families.

Agency for Health Care Policy and Research Publications Clearinghouse
P.O. Box 8547
Silver Spring, MD 90907
(800) 358-9295
A clearinghouse that provides information on cataract to consumers.

American Academy of Ophthalmology
655 Beach Street
San Francisco, CA 94109
(415) 561-8500
www.eyenet.org
This leading professional organization offers a vast array of information on eye and vision problems, such as low vision, glaucoma, cataracts, and macular degeneration. To obtain free patient information brochures, send a self-addressed, stamped envelope and note the topic(s) desired to the address listed.

American Autoimmune Related Diseases Association, Inc.
22100 Gratiot Avenue
E. Detroit, MI 48021
(800) 598-4668 (literature request)
(810) 776-3900
www.aarda.org

Provides information on autoimmune diseases that can affect eyesight, such as Graves' disease, Sjögren's syndrome, and multiple sclerosis.

American Council of the Blind
1155 15th Street, N.W., Suite 720
Washington, D.C. 20005
(800) 424-8666
(202) 467-5081
www.acb.org
Offers a variety of services to the visually impaired; emphasizes employment opportunities.

American Diabetes Association
1701 North Beauregard Street
Alexandria, VA 22311
(703) 549-1500
www.diabetes.org
Provides information on diabetes, eye care, and diabetes-related vision disorders, such as diabetic retinopathy.

American Foundation for the Blind
11 Penn Plaza, Suite 300
New York, NY 10001
(800) AFB-LINE (800-232-5463)
(212) 502-7600
www.afb.org
Serves as a national clearinghouse for information about blindness and visual impairment. Provides referrals for patients to low-vision centers.

American Macular Degeneration Foundation
P.O. Box 515
Northampton, MA 01061-0515
(413) 268-7660
www.macular.org
Offers health tips for consumers on the prevention and treatment of macular degeneration.

American Optometric Association
243 North Lindbergh Boulevard
St. Louis, MO 63141
(314) 991-4100
www.aoanet.org
Provides information on low vision and other eye problems.

American Society of Cataract and Refractive Surgery
4000 Legato Rd., Suite 850
Fairfax, VA 22033
(703) 591-2220
www.ascrs.org
Provides information on the latest advances in cataract extraction and surgical procedures to correct optical errors.

Association for Macular Diseases, Inc.
P.O. Box 220154
Great Neck, NY 11022-0154
(212) 605-3719
www.macula.org
A national support group for those affected by macular degeneration; offers education and information on macular diseases through seminars, newsletters and a hotline. Offers coun-

seling to patients and their families. Publishes a quarterly newsletter, *Eyes Only*. Membership: $20. Send a self-addressed, stamped envelope for information.

Associated Services for the Blind
919 Walnut Street, 2nd Floor
Philadelphia, PA 19107
(215) 627-0600
www.libertynet.org/asbinfo/
Offers personal adjustment to blindness training and orientation and mobility training. Offers computer training using adaptive devices.

Council of Citizens with Low Vision International
(800) 733-2258
(317) 254-1332
Serves as an advocacy group for the visually impaired and provides information on low vision technology.

Diabetic Retinopathy Foundation
350 North LaSalle
Suite 800
Chicago, IL 60610
http://www.retinopathy.org
Provides information on diabetic retinopathy.

EyeCare America—National Eye Care Project
(800) 222-EYES (800) 222-3937
www.eyenet.org/public/pi/service/necp.html
Coordinated by the American Academy of Ophthalmology, this program provides free eye exams and medical treatment for

U.S. citizens age sixty-five and older who haven't had access to an ophthalmologist during the past three years. The program is cosponsored by the Knight's Templar Eye Foundation and state ophthalmological societies.

Glaucoma Research Foundation
200 Pine St., Suite 200
San Francisco, CA 94104
(800) 826-6693
(415) 986-3162
www.glaucoma.org
Provides educational materials on glaucoma, including a free quarterly newsletter, *Gleams,* and *Understanding and Living with Glaucoma,* a resource guide for people with glaucoma and their families.

International Society of Refractive Surgery
1180 Springs Centre South Blvd., Suite 116
Altamonte Springs, FL 32714
www.isrs.org
Provides patient information on laser vision correction and other surgical treatments for refractive errors of the eye, such as nearsightedness and farsightedness.

Knights Templar Eye Foundation
5097 North Elston Avenue
Suite 100
Chicago, IL 60630-2460
www.knightstemplar.org/ktef
This foundation provides financial assistance for eye surgery for those who aren't able to pay or cannot receive adequate assis-

tance from current government agencies or similar sources. They also cosponsor the Foundation of the American Academy of Ophthalmology's National Eye Care project.

Lighthouse International
111 East 59th St., 12th floor
New York, NY 10022
(800) 829-0500
(212) 821-9200
www.lighthouse.org
Provides educational materials on age-related vision problems and referrals to vision and rehabilitation agencies. Call for a catalog of nonoptical aids for daily living.

Lions Clubs International
300 22nd Street
Oak Brook, IL 60523-8842
(630) 571-5466 (national office)
www.lionsclubs.org
This organization provides patient education materials on glaucoma and other eye diseases, as well as financial assistance to individuals for eye care through local Lions Clubs. There are Lions Clubs in most areas; services vary from club to club. Check your telephone book for the telephone number and address of your local club.

Low Vision Gateway
www.lowvision.org
A web site sponsored by The Internet Low Vision Society and the Low Vision Centers of Indiana dedicated to providing information and resources for people with low vision and their fami-

lies. Contains links to information on low-vision specialists, low-vision aids, and organizations that provide support and assistance.

Macular Degeneration International
6700 N. Oracle Rd., Suite 121
Tucson, AZ 85704
(520) 797-2525
www.maculardegeneration.org
Offers educational seminars and consumer materials for people affected by juvenile and age-related macular degeneration. Annual membership fee ($25) includes resource book, twice-yearly newsletter, and a complimentary newsletter for family members.

Maryland Society for Sight
1313 West Old Cold Spring Lane
Baltimore, MD 21209
(410) 243-2020
www.mdsocietyforsight.org
This nonprofit health organization works to prevent blindness and preserve sight for all Marylanders, regardless of geographic or economic limitations. Programs include adult vision screenings and volunteers for the visually impaired.

Mission Cataract USA
(800) 343-7265
This program, coordinated by the Volunteer Eye Surgeons' Association, provides free cataract surgery for people of all ages who otherwise can't afford it. Surgeries are scheduled yearly on one day, usually in May.

National Association for Visually Handicapped
22 W. 21st Street, 6th Floor
New York, NY 10010
(212) 889-3141
An information clearinghouse for services available to the partially sighted; conducts self-help groups. Provides information on large-print books, textbooks, and educational tools. Publishes a quarterly newsletter and has a large-print loan library with over 7,000 titles. Sells a variety of optical aids for the visually impaired.

National Eye Institute (NEI)
of the National Institutes of Health
2020 Vision Place
Bethesda, MD 20892-3655
(301) 496-5248
www.nei.nih.gov
The NEI supports research on eye disease and the visual system. The NEI can send you free brochures on eye disorders if you call or write.

National Institute of Diabetes and Digestive and Kidney Diseases
1 Information Way
Bethesda, MD 20892-3560
(301) 654-3327
www.niddk.nih.gov
Offers easy-to-read publications for consumers on preventing and treating diabetes.

National Institute on Aging
Building 31, Room 5C27

31 Center Drive, MSC 2292

Bethesda, MD 20892

(301) 496-1752

www.nih.gov/nia

Offers health information on age-related eye diseases, and taking care of your eyes as you get older.

New Eyes for the Needy

549 Millburn Avenue

P.O. Box 332

Short Hills, New Jersey 07078-0332

(973) 376-4903

This organization provides vouchers for the purchase of new prescription eyeglasses.

National Federation of the Blind

1800 Johnson Street

Baltimore, MD 21230

(410) 659-9314

www.nfb.org

Provides a variety of services for the visually impaired.

National Library Service for the Blind and Visually Handicapped

1291 Taylor Street, NW

Washington, D.C. 20542

(800) 424-8567

Provides free library services to people with vision problems, and offers Braille and large-print materials, recorded books, and periodicals.

Prevent Blindness America
500 East Remington Rd.
Schaumburg, IL 60173-5611
(800) 331-2020
www.preventblindness.org
Provides fact sheets, brochures, and information on eye safety, eye care, vision screening, and eye ailments as well as a web site forum for patients and consumers who wish to discuss eye problems with others in similar situations.

Prevention of Blindness Society of the Metropolitan Area
1775 Church Street, NW
Washington, D.C. 20036
(202) 234-1010
www.youreyes.org
A nonprofit organization that seeks to prevent needless vision loss among those in the Washington, D.C. metropolitan area. Sponsors vision screening, eye health, and safety-education programs, the Macular Degeneration Network, and provides eye care to the poor and homeless.

Resources for Rehabilitation
33 Bedford Street, Suite 19A
Lexington, MA 02420
(781) 862-6455
www.rfr.org
Offers training programs for the public on coping with low vision.

Sjögren's Syndrome Foundation
366 North Broadway

Jericho, NY 11753

(800) 475-6473

(516) 933-6365

www.sjogrens.com

Provides support and education for people with Sjögren's syndrome and publishes *The Sjögren's Syndrome Handbook* and the newsletter *Moisture Seekers*.

The Glaucoma Foundation

116 John Street, Ste. 1605

New York, NY 10038

(800) GLAUCOMA (800-452-8266)

(212) 285-0080

http://www.glaucoma-foundation.org/info

A not-for-profit organization dedicated to glaucoma research and public education. Offers numerous information resources for patients and their families, including patient education materials on glaucoma prevention and treatment.

The Medicine Program

P.O. Box 4182

Poplar Bluff, Missouri 63902-4182

(573) 996-7300

www.themedicineprogram.com

This program assists people to enroll in one or more of the many patient-assistance programs that provide free prescription medicine to those in need. Patients must meet the sponsor's criteria. The program is conducted in cooperation with the patient's doctor.

U.S. Department of Education

Rehabilitation Services Administration

330 C Street, S.W., Room 3229

Washington, DC 20202-2741

(202) 205-9320

Provides training in skills of routine daily living, travel, communication, adaptive devices, low-vision services, family and peer counseling. Programs available in every state, accessible through each state agency for the blind.

U.S. Food and Drug Administration

5600 Fishers Lane

Rockville, MD 20857-0001

(888) INFO-FDA (888-463-6332)

www.fda.gov

Provides objective information for consumers on LASIK surgery, including a glossary of terms, a checklist of issues for patients to consider, and questions to ask the eye doctor before undergoing the procedure.

Vision Community Services

A Division of the Massachusetts Association for the Blind

23A Elm Street

Watertown, MA 02472

(800) 852-3029 (MA only)

(617) 962-4232

Provides local, national, and international resources to consumers and their families. Offers a wide variety of cooking equipment, recreational, and household items specially designed or adapted for use by those with vision loss. A catalog of these assistance devices is available in large print, audiocassette, and on computer disk.

VISIONS/Services for the Blind and Visually Impaired
500 Greenwich Street, 3rd Floor
New York, NY 10013-1354
(888) 245-8333
(212) 625-1616
www.visionsvcb.org
Offers free services for those over age fifty-five with severe vision problems. Services include self-help study kits, counseling, vision rehabilitation training, computer workshops, and an information center.

VISION USA
(800) 766-4466
Coordinated by the American Optometric Association, the program provides free eye care to uninsured low-income workers and their families. Screening for the program takes place in January of each year, with exams provided later in the year.

Index

Page numbers in *italics* refer to illustrations.